The Mini Neurology Series
Volume 2:
Carpal Tunnel Syndrome
By
Britt Talley Daniel MD

Discover other titles by this author at
http://www.britttalleydanielmdauthor.com
Migraine, second edition
Transient Global Amnesia
The Mini Neurology Series: Volume 1 Migraine
Volume 2 Carpal Tunnel Syndrome
Volume 3 Panic Disorder
Volume 4 Essential Tremor
Titanic: Answer from the Deep
The Mysteries of MacArthur Donne:
Book 1 And If Thine Eye Offend Thee
Book 2 The Case of the Organic Chemist
Book 3 The Spanish Flu 1918

Dedication

Carpal tunnel syndrome is the wrist/hand problem of now. Carpal tunnel syndrome is a product of the computer age and is found in schools where students write, type, or text notes all day long. It's in the office with the employee who types or uses ten key equipment. It's in the kitchen with the person who scrubs or cleans floors, or out on the street with the jackhammer operator.

This book is dedicated to all medical personnel who care for and those affected by the numb, the weak, the painful limbs from carpal tunnel syndrome.

Table of Contents

Chapter 1 Anatomy

<u>Median nerve pathway</u>
The median nerve originates from C5, C6, C7, and T1 located neurons in the cervical spinal cord. The processes of these roots pass through the brachial plexus as the upper and lower trunks and then unite in mid-shoulder forming the medial cord of the brachial plexus. At the lateral or outer portion of the shoulder the medial and lateral cords of the brachial plexus merge to give off the median nerve near the head of the humerus which passes through the axillary fossa and then travels down the upper arm next to the humerus and under the biceps muscle. At the ventral side of the elbow, the anticubital space, the median nerve becomes superficial and gives off its first muscular branch, the pronator teres which functions to turn the arm over so the palm would lie flat on a table.

The median nerve next provides all the muscles in the forearm which contract the tips of the fingers and small muscles separating the index and third fingers except the branch to flexor carpi ulnaris which is innervated by the ulnar nerve. In the upper forearm the median nerve gives off the nerve to the tip of the thumb, the flexor pollicis longus, and then proceeds down the forearm. At the wrist the median nerve pierces the carpal tunnel and divides into its sensory, motor, and autonomic branches. The motor fibers usually innervate the muscle that holds the thumb apart from the palm, the abductor pollicis brevis, the opponens pollicis, the muscle that brings the thumb to the little finger, the radial half of the flexor pollicis brevis, and the lumbricals to the index and middle fingers.

It is common for the ulnar and median nerves to overlap their supply to the flexor pollicis brevis muscle. Depending on the amount of cross-innervation, opposition of the thumb (movement out of the plane of the palm) can occur due to muscles supplied by the ulnar nerve. Also, the same motion can occur through traces of the abductor pollicis longus innervated by the radial nerve. Therefore, thumb oppositional movement cannot be interpreted as evidence of function of median nerve innervated thenar muscles.

The palmar sensory cutaneous branch of the median nerve comes off the median nerve immediately above the transverse carpal ligament, passes through a short tunnel within the transverse carpal tunnel, and innervates sensation over the thenar eminence. Damage to this branch produces paresthesias over the thenar eminence and is indicative of median neuropathy above the carpal tunnel. This nerve can be injured by a transverse incision at the wrist during carpal tunnel decompression and by ganglion resulting from blunt trauma to the wrist. It also supplies the skin of the palm. The palmar sensory cutaneous branch does not pass through the carpal tunnel and therefore the palm is not affected in CTS. Sensory fibers constitute 94% of the median nerve and are usually the first to be affected by compression in the carpal tunnel.

Median autonomic fibers go through the superficial palmar arch and join the digital vessels of the palm, index, long fingers, and radial half of the ring finger through the digital nerves. Autonomic dysfunction can cause anhydrosis (lack of sweating), red or purple skin from vasodilatation, or hypohydrosis (reduced sweating).

Carpal tunnel anatomy

The mystery and the agony and everything that this book is about occurs as the median nerve passes through the carpal tunnel. The carpal tunnel syndrome is the most common and familiar type of median nerve entrapment, making up 90% of all entrapment neuropathies. An entrapment neuropathy is a chronic focal compressive neuropathy caused by pressure increase inside non-flexible anatomical structures. The carpal tunnel is a tight, restricted osseo-ligamentous passage at the wrist made up of the carpal bones on the deep or posterior side and the transverse carpal ligament, also called the flexor retinaculum, on the front or anterior side. The walls of the carpal tunnel are unyielding and any encroachment on the enclosed space, such as by fracture or dislocation of a carpal bone, Colles' fracture, swelling of ligaments, or osteoarthritic changes cause constriction of the median nerve fibers. Also, swelling of the carpal tunnel contents due to local pathologic processes of systemic disease can constrict more yielding elements of the tunnel, such as the median nerve.

Nine flexor tendons, two extending to each finger and one to the thumb, pass through the carpal tunnel with the median nerve. The tendons of flexor pollicis longus, flexor digitorum sublimis, and flexor digitorum profundus pass through the tunnel. The thenar branch of the median nerve usually passes through a separate tunnel through the transverse carpal ligament. The median nerve is sometimes accompanied by a persistent median artery, but always by the tiny microscopic arteries, called the vasa nervourum, the arteries that supply blood to the median nerve itself. A persistent median artery is found in one hand or unilaterally in 20 % of persons and in both hands or bilaterally in 6 %. A persistent median artery, probably by occupying space in the carpal tunnel, may be a cause of carpal tunnel syndrome.

The transverse carpal ligament is a strong, fibrous band of tissue closing off the carpal tunnel. In cases of the syndrome that come to surgery, it is the transverse carpal ligament that the surgeon cuts to release the median nerve. Persons with carpal tunnel syndrome usually have abnormalities of the tunnel which predisposes them to develop carpal tunnel symptoms from constriction and compromise of the median nerve.

Variation in Median fibers

Median sensory fibers in hand classically innervate the palmar thumb, index, middle finger and the radial portion of the ring finger in 75% of patients. However, there may be many variations in the sensory innervation, such as an "all median sensory hand" where all of the fingers and the thumb receive sensation from the median nerve and the patient may complain of numbness or tingling in all the fingers and the thumb. Also fibers in the median nerve at the elbow may cross over to the ulnar nerve in the forearm in 15 % to 30 % of normal persons.

This cross over feature is called the Martin Gruber anastomosis which is important mainly in the EMG lab where it may confuse the electromyographer and is discussed in more detail in Chapter 6.

Median Nerve

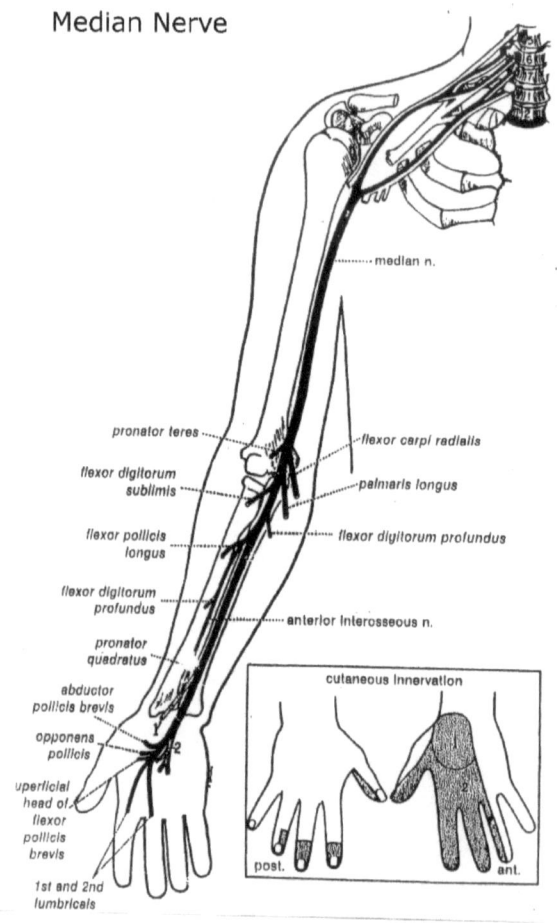

median n.

pronator teres

flexor digitorum
sublimis

flexor pollicis
longus

flexor digitorum
profundus

pronator
quadratus

abductor
pollicis brevis

opponens
pollicis

uperficial
head of
flexor
pollicis
brevis

1st and 2nd
lumbricals

flexor carpi radialis

palmaris longus

flexor digitorum profundus

anterior interosseous n.

cutaneous innervation

post.

ant.

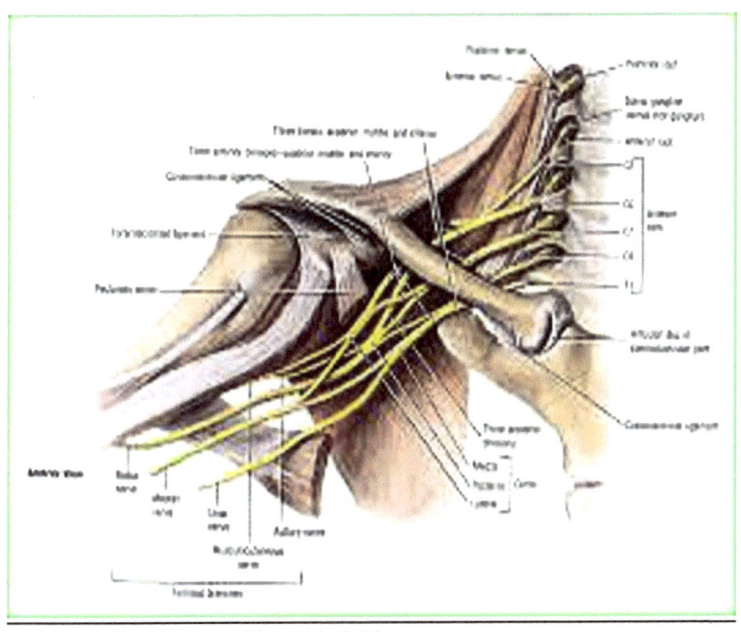

Brachial Plexus

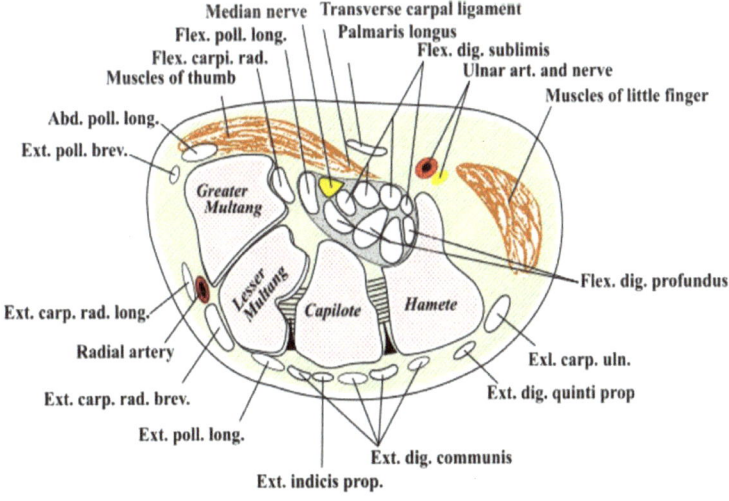

Median nerve · Transverse carpal ligament
Flex. poll. long. · Palmaris longus
Flex. carpi. rad. · Flex. dig. sublimis
Muscles of thumb · Ulnar art. and nerve
Muscles of little finger
Abd. poll. long.
Ext. poll. brev.
Greater Multang
Flex. dig. profundus
Lesser Multang
Capilote · Hamete
Ext. carp. rad. long.
Radial artery
Exl. carp. uln.
Ext. carp. rad. brev.
Ext. dig. quinti prop
Ext. poll. long.
Ext. dig. communis
Ext. indicis prop.

Cross Section of Carpal Tunnel

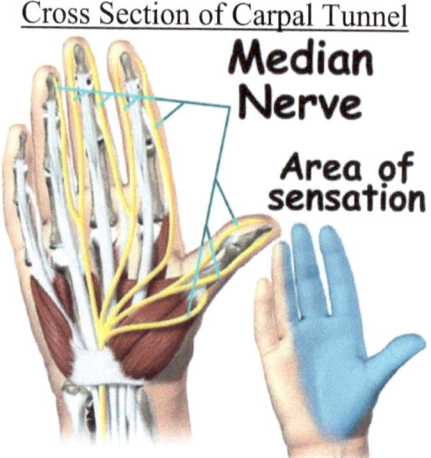

Median Nerve

Area of sensation

Median Nerve Distribution

Chapter 2 Symptoms

<u>Median fibers</u>
The median nerve carries four types of fibers through the tunnel into the hand: motor fibers providing muscular power to the thumb and fingers, sensory fibers for touch and pressure, sensory fibers for pain and temperature, and small autonomic fibers which provide vasomotor control of the microvasculature and activation of the sweat glands. Clinically, and from the patient's point of view, if the motor fibers are involved then the patient complains of weakness of grip or of dropping things from the hand. If the sensory fibers for touch are involved, then the patient complains of "numbness and tingling" or a "dead" or a "pins and needles" type feeling. If the sensory fibers for pain and temperature are involved, then the patient complains of pain which may be burning or hot or even cold. The pain of carpal tunnel syndrome can be very severe and level 10 on a scale of 1-10. If the autonomic fibers which go to the small blood vessels and provide sweating in the hand are involved, then the patient may complain of swelling, redness, fingertip ulcers, or edema.

In 2002 the American Association of Electrodiagnostic Medicine, American Academy of Neurology, and the American Academy of Physical Medicine and Rehabilitation published "Practice Parameter: electrodiagnostic studies in carpal tunnel syndrome." This paper expanded the first CTS Literature Review published in 1993. Regarding clinical symptoms of CTS, the document listed inclusion criteria:

Sensory symptoms (numbness and/or tingling) in at least 2 of digits 1, 2, 3, and 4 for at least 1 month. The sensory symptoms may be intermittent or constant, but if constant, there must have been a period of time during which the symptoms were intermittent. The numbness and tingling may be accompanied by pain, but pain alone is not sufficient to meet this first inclusion criteria.

Sensory symptoms (numbness and/or tingling) aggravated by at least 1 of the following: sleep, sustained hand or arm positioning, or repetitive actions of the hand.

Sensory symptoms (numbness and/or tingling) mitigated by at least 1 of the following: changes in hand posture, shaking the hand, or use of a wrist splint.

If pain is present, the wrist, hand, and finger pain is greater than elbow, shoulder, or neck pain if there is pain in any or all of those locations.

This document also suggested exclusion criteria:

Sensory symptoms exclusive or predominantly in the D5 (little finger) (ulnar neuropathy).

Neck pain or shoulder pain

preceded the paresthesia in the digits (cervical radiculopathy and/or brachial plexopathy). Numbness and/or tingling in the feet which preceded or accompanied the sensory symptoms in the hands (polyneuropathy). Findings on the problem focused history and physical examination which indicate an explanation for the sensory symptoms which is more probable than CTS, for example, digital neuropathy, median nerve pathology proximal to the carpal tunnel, ulnar neuropathy, radial neuropathy, brachial plexopathy, cervical radiculopathy, spinal cord, brainstem or brain pathology, or a polyneuropathy.

Pathophysiology

Elevated pressure and compression causes focal disturbances in myelin and paranodal demyelination. It has been shown that focal compression of the median nerve in healthy persons resulted in axonal depolarization. This results in blocked nerve transmission (neuropraxia) which if chronic, can affect the blood flow to the endoneural capillary. This produces changes in the blood-nerve barrier and endoneural edema. A cycle of venous congestion, ischemia, and local metabolic changes occurs which results in axonal degeneration, macrophage attraction, release of inflammatory cytokines, nitric oxide, and a "chemical neuritis."

Flexion and extension movements, work overuse, and vibration can set off these pathological changes. In America 8-10 million workers are exposed to the vibration of power tools. An experiment of vibration injury in rat tails found thinning and loss of endothelial cells and activated platelets in the exposed subendothelial tissue, indications of denuding of the arterial endothelium.

Development of symptoms

Usually, the sensory fibers for touch are the first involved with development of early symptoms, likely because the sensory fibers are very small and sensitive to pressure which causes ischemia in the nerve fibers themselves. Then next, as time goes on, the patient may complain of swelling of the hand, indicating involvement of the tiny autonomic fibers. Later pain develops and there may be weakness of grip, such as holding a glass or a pan. Weakness of grip leads to dropping things, another late, but common symptom.

Older age presentation

A common presentation is the older patient, aged 65-80, who comes in for weakness of the thumb base and some mild hand pain. Most of these patients, when studied clinically have thenar atrophy and weakness, normal provocative tests, such as the Tinel sign or Phalen maneuver, and the development of median sensory neuropathy indicated by lack of pin sensation over the volar median fingers to the palm. Sometimes on close questioning the patient may recall having nocturnal or driving induced paresthesiae years previously, but many don't recall this. Electrodiagnostic study of such patients usually shows no median sensory response, markedly prolonged median distal motor latencies (6-10 msec), and denervation on needle exam of the abductor pollicis brevis muscle.

Localization of sensory fibers

Note should be made that the sensory fibers for touch can be well located by the brain. A demonstration of this would be a person's ability to tell which of their fingers were touched by someone else with their eyes closed. Human beings are readily able to tell which of their fingers has been touched by someone else with their eyes closed. However, the fibers that carry pain and temperature are not well located by the brain. This anatomical fact carries with it the problem of the patient localizing where in their body the pain from carpal tunnel syndrome originates. Even though carpal tunnel syndrome is due to median nerve compression in the wrist, the pain may be "referred" to another part of the body. Pain from carpal tunnel syndrome may be referred to the forearm or upper arm. This is a source of great clinical confusion and results in tests at the "wrong" location in the body, such as X-rays of the arm or shoulder or CAT or MRI scans of the cervical region looking for a cervical disc when the clinical problem is at the wrist and due to median neuropathy from carpal tunnel syndrome.

The brain can't localize deep pain well. Another example of referred pain would be a person with a heart attack or myocardial infarction involving the heart, which is in the chest, causing pain in the left arm, shoulder, chin, or even the dorsal chest. The pain is not coming from the left arm but from the chest where the heart is located. A herniated cervical disc usually causes pain in the back of the upper arm, in the triceps area, or laterally under the shoulder blade, when the problem is actually coming from the compressed nerve root at the dorsal cervical spine area.

Also the phrase "sciatica" which is actually an anatomic misnomer and inaccurate, denotes pain in the back of the hip or thigh from a pinched nerve, when the problem is actually coming from a "pinched nerve" or lumbar disc herniation located low in the back near the spinal cord. The sciatic nerve is made up of fibers from the lumbosacral plexus comprising the fourth and fifth lumbar roots and sacral roots 1,2,3. It is named the "sciatic nerve" after it receives fibers from the lumbosacral plexus at the level of the head of the femur after which it descends down the leg and gives off motor and sensory fibers to the peroneal and tibial nerves. The anatomical misnomer is that a herniated lumbar disc strikes the root just adjacent to the cord in the lower back, not at the head of the femur, where the sciatic nerve originates, a distance of some 10 cm away.

In a similar fashion the numbness and tingling of carpal tunnel syndrome, although originating in the wrist, may seem to the patient to be located in the fingers and thumb, the hand, forearm, or upper arm. These factors confuse patients suffering the symptoms and doctors who are trying to figure out what is wrong.

<u>Other Median nerve syndromes</u>

Other syndromes involving the median nerve are very rare and include anatomical involvement at the anticubital fossa area called the pronator teres syndrome, where the nerve is trapped between the two heads of the pronator teres muscle, or the anterior interosseous syndrome due to compression of the median nerve in the forearm above the carpal tunnel.

Thoracic Outlet Syndrome (TOS)

This is a complex clinical syndrome which includes:

    Vascular subtypes
        Arterial vascular TOS
        Venous vascular TOS
    Neurologic subtypes
        True neurologic TOS
        Nonspecific TOS
    Neurovascular subtypes
        Traumatic neurovascular TOS
        Nonspecific TOS
    Musculoskeletal subtypes
        Nonspecific TOS

Thoracic Outlet Syndrome refers to a heterogenous group of disorders all of which have in common compression of one or more of the neurovascular elements at some point within the thoracic outlet. Mark Ferrante reviewed "The Thoracic Outlet Syndromes" in 2011 in *Muscle & Nerve*. Many of these diverse syndromes may cause symptoms of pain, tingling, swelling, weakness, and muscle atrophy. TOS involves various components of the brachial plexus, the blood vessels, or both at different sites between the base of the neck and the axilla. The arterial form is caused by compression of the subclavian artery, the venous form is caused by compression of the subclavian vein, and the neurologic form is caused by brachial plexus compression. Combined neurovascular TOS is usually traumatic.

True Neurologic TOS is rare with a prevalence of 1/1,000,000. Most affected persons are women who are young to middle-aged. For every 20,000-80,000 individuals with a cervical rib 1 will have true neurologic TOS. The cause was first reported by Thomas and Cushing in 1903 as due to stretching of the inferior elements of the supraclavicular brachial plexus by a taut band extending from the first thoracic rib to a bony anomaly at C7 which is either a small cervical rib or an elongated transverse process.

Motor symptoms predominate clinically, and the patients present with intrinsic hand muscle weakness and wasting. Weakness may involve thenar, ulnar and medial forearm muscles. Sensory abnormalities of aching and paresthesia predominate along the medial forearm. X-ray of the cervical spine may show the cervical rib or transverse process while cervical CAT and MRI scanning may be helpful in ruling out a lower C8 or T1 radiculopathy, but the elastic band causing true neurologic TOS is not well seen by CAT or MRI scanning.

On the Electrodiagnostic Exam (EDX) the ulnar and medial antebrachial cutaneous Sensory Nerve Action Potentials (SNAPs) are absent, the median, ulnar, and distal radial Compound Motor Action Potentials (CMAPs) are abnormally low in amplitude, and the needle exam shows a reduced number of long duration, large amplitude, units with rare fibrillation. TOS causes such chronic neurologic damage mostly in the abductor pollicis brevis, and to a lesser degree in medial and distal forearm muscles innervated by the ulnar and median nerve such as the first dorsal interosseous and flexor pollicis longus muscles.

There is no role for conservative management of true neurologic TOS and patients should always be treated by surgical cutting of the fibrous band via a supraclavicular approach.

Carpal tunnel syndrome symptoms

Carpal tunnel syndrome (CTS) is the most common compression neuropathy of the upper limb. The symptoms usually start gradually and common initial symptoms are itching numbness, "pins and needles", tingling, burning, a dead sensation, and a lack of feeling which is usually in the fingers and hand. The fingers may feel "useless and swollen" even though no swelling may be noted. The symptoms often appear in one or both hands during the night because many people sleep with flexed wrists. Some patients can localize the symptoms to be worse or only present in the median innervated digits (thumb, index, middle finger, median half of the ring finger). Others can't do this. Sometimes the numbness seems to be in the wrist, forearm, or upper arm. Numbness or pain may worsen while using the involved hand especially in gripping something or bending the wrist. The hand may get numb at night, awakening the patient, or while performing some job with their hand, such as writing, driving, typing, using the mouse, or hair dryer. The patient may find their arm is only comfortable when lying straight out at their side in bed, but not in their lap, or above their head. The patient may have to go through elaborate arm positioning in bed before they go to sleep so their hand doesn't bother them during the night.

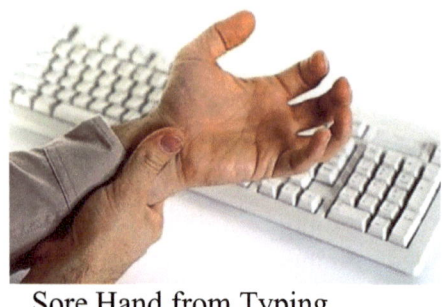

Sore Hand from Typing

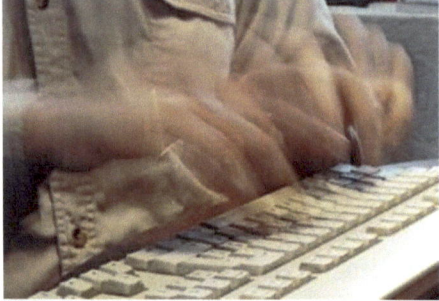

Rapid Typing

Persons with carpal tunnel syndrome may awaken feeling the need to "shake out" or "flip" the hand or wrist. As the symptoms worsen tingling may occur during the day. Some patients report an electric "funny bone" type sensation with use of the hand, such as pushing down with the thumb with the hand flexed to open a car door. Pain is typically aching, burning, or throbbing. Some patients complain of weakness in the hand. The patient may have trouble with simple hand movements such as hair brushing or holding a fork. They may accidentally drop objects due to reduced pinched strength between the thumb and first finger or while doing simple tasks such as opening a jar or using a screwdriver. This is usually weakness involving grip of the fingers or thumb, for acts such as holding a glass, or a heavy pan between the thumb and flexor fingers. Late in CTS there may be atrophy (wasting, or lack of bulk) of the muscles at the base of the thumb. Autonomic neurologic symptoms may occur also, such as swelling or redness of the hands, dryness, and changes in nail growth. Ultimately some patients develop median sensory neuropathy and are unable to tell hot or cold with their fingers by touch. They can't identify different coins or keys in their pocket without looking. Rare patients present with chronic erythema involving the volar thumb, index, middle, and half of the ring finger which later results in typical CTS symptoms of pain, numbness, and weakness.

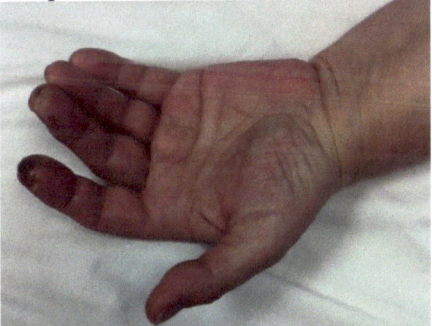

Red Fingers and Distal Necrosis
Stages of Carpal Tunnel Syndrome

Some writers have described progressive carpal tunnel syndrome as occurring in 3 stages.

Stage 1 The patient has frequent awakenings during the night with symptoms of a swollen, numb hand. There may be severe pain that radiates from the wrist to the shoulder and annoying tingling of the hand and fingers. Hand shaking usually relieves the symptoms. Although still numb and swollen on awakening in the morning, the symptoms resolve quickly within minutes and the patient goes on with his day.

Stage 2 The symptoms come during the day, usually when the patient is in the same position or performs repeated movements with their hand or wrist. Reading the newspaper or holding a book or typing or using the mouse may set off symptoms. Transient numbness progresses to anesthesia and the patient is unable to feel his fingers anymore or he may drop items from his hands because he can't feel them or his thenar muscles, opposing the thumb are weak.

Stage 3 In this final stage thenar atrophy and thumb opposition muscle acts such has holding a glass, or a pan are evident. Sensory symptoms may decrease as aching in the thenar, forearm, upper arm, and shoulder progress.

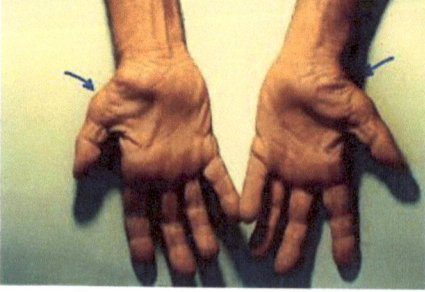

Severe Thenar Atrophy

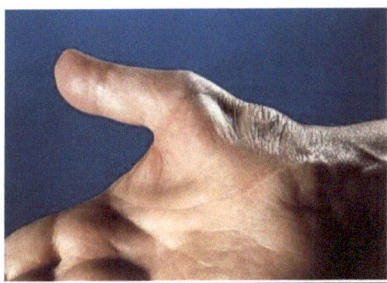

Side View Thenar Atrophy

Also, paradoxically, many patients have short lived symptoms lasting months to half a year and then their symptoms clear up and they are okay.
Pregnancy related carpal tunnel syndrome usually clears with delivery of the baby and the weight loss, usually through fluid diuresis, that occurs over the next several months.

My experience is that many patients that I am seeing now for typical carpal tunnel syndrome symptoms often forget the symptoms they had five or ten years ago. These symptoms brought them to their internist or family practice doctor who advised them to get a splint which they used for a month or two and then the symptoms completely resolved. Many of these patients still have their splints but seem to not really have understood how the splint worked or that their symptoms related to carpal tunnel syndrome.

Also there are the patients who Google their symptoms and fear they have some more severe neurologic illness like multiple sclerosis which also causes numbness but a very different clinical course and distribution of symptoms.

Familial Carpal Tunnel Syndrome

Phalen stated in 1966, "Many patients offer the information that their parents or grandparents had similar complaints. There is probably some sort of predisposition to carpal tunnel syndrome."' A significant family history of CTS is found in many patients with confirmed CTS. This may relate to personal characteristics such as age, wrist depth/width ratio, carpal ligament thickness, and height and weight of individual members in a family. Family here refers to 2 or 3 generations of members. A prospective study investigating the prevalence and significance of a positive family history of carpal tunnel syndrome found 75/253 women and 40/168 men with confirmed CTS had at least one relative with symptoms of, or surgery for, carpal tunnel syndrome. The same study of 84 patients with previous carpal tunnel surgery had a positive family history of 39.3%. However, one must always remember that a family history of any medical problem is always second-hand information.

CTS questionaires

There are a number of published questionnaires used for the diagnosis of carpal tunnel syndrome. The American Association of Orthopedic Surgeons in their publication: "AAOS Clinical Guidelines on the Treatment of Carpal Tunnel Syndrome" recommend the following:

Boston Carpal Tunnel Questionaire
DASH—Disabilities of the Arm, Shoulder, and Hand
MHQ—Michigan Hand Outcomes Questionaire
Patient Evaluation Measure—hand
Other medical hand conditions
Thumb/finger Osteoarthritis

Since carpal tunnel syndrome comes with ageing and use of the hand, many persons with carpal tunnel syndrome also have osteoarthritis of the fingers or the base of the thumb. Osteoarthritis causes swelling, thumb movement pain, curvature of the fingers, or the development of an osteophyte or bone spur. With osteoarthritis of the fingers or thumb there may be tenderness; that is the digits are sensitive to pressure or movement. This pain may be confused with the pain of carpal tunnel syndrome which does not cause tenderness. That is, with CTS, palpation or pressure on the digits or thumb doesn't hurt. Carpal tunnel pain comes with flexed or extended positions of the wrist or with use of the hands. Osteoarthritis of the thumb base may be treated with rest, local cortisone injection, or surgery.

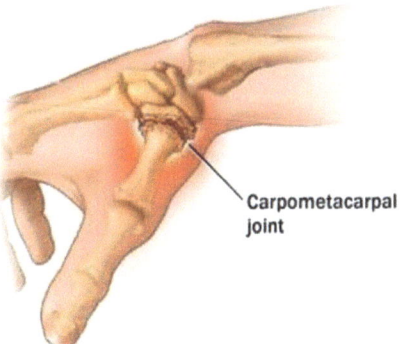

Carpometacarpal joint

Thumb-base Osteoarthritis

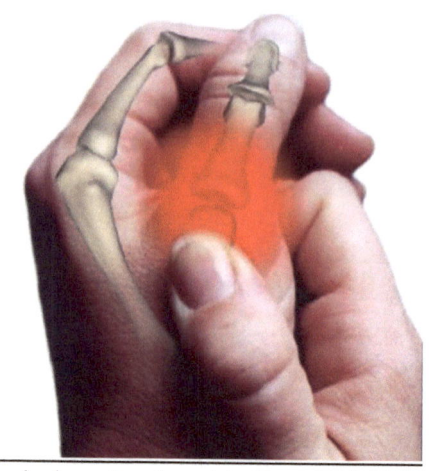

Palpation induced pain with Osteoarthritis.

Trigger finger

Also, some patients may develop a "trigger finger" which is also called stenosing tenosynovitis. This is a tendon sheath problem which makes flexion of a digit feel stuck or slow (as a bump or enlargement on the tendon tries to slip through the tendon sheath). Symptoms of "trigger finger" commonly occur in the palm, involve the tendons of the 3rd or 4th digits and are different from carpal tunnel syndrome. Trigger finger may be associated with CTS and can be treated by an orthopedic surgeon with cortisone injection or surgery.

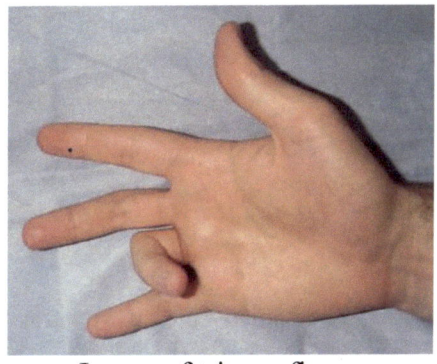

Image of trigger finger

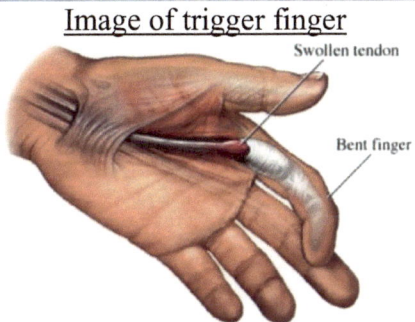

Swollen tendon

Bent finger

Red swollen tendon sheath

De Quervain's disease

Another orthopedic condition sometimes confused with carpal tunnel syndrome is de Quervain's disease, named after the Swiss surgeon, Fritz de Quervain, who described in 1895 a syndrome of pain, tenderness, swelling, and difficulty gripping with the fingers. This is a dorsal thumb located problem due to tendon sheath inflammation, perhaps related to repetitive strain injury, of the extensor pollicis brevis and abductor pollicis longus muscles. Diagnosis is secured by a positive Finkelstein's test which is performed by the physician grasping the thumb and ulnar deviating the hand sharply. Sharp pain on the distal dorsal radius an inch below the wrist makes the diagnosis. Treatment is rest, splint immobilization, and local cortisone injection.

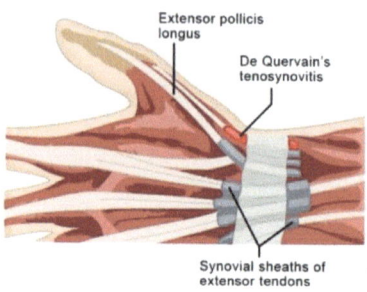

Extensor pollicis longus

De Quervain's tenosynovitis

Synovial sheaths of extensor tendons

© Sinew Therapeutics

Tendon involved with De Quervain's disease.

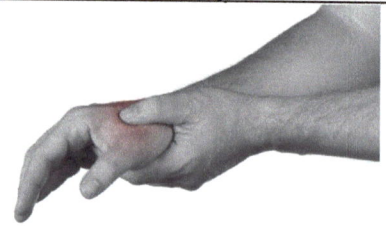

Palpation pain with De Quervain's disease

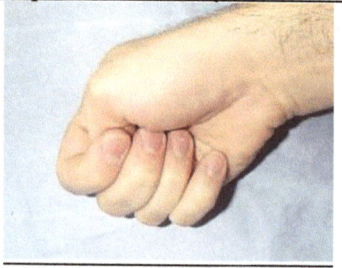

Finklestein's Test

Raynaud's phenomenon/disease

Patients may develop Raynaud's phenomenon (not associated with autoimmune disease) or Raynaud's disease (associated with connective tissue or autoimmune disease, such as systemic lupus erythematosus, or rheumatoid arthritis). Both conditions consist of symptoms of the ears, nose, fingers, or toes that occur after exposure to a cold environment or stress such as winter exposure of the digits to cold by holding a snowball or ice cube or stressful life events. Cold exposure causes vasoconstriction and ischemia of the small blood vessels in the digits. This may give symptoms of: cold fingers and toes, color changes in the skin, turning white, blue, or red, numbness and tingling of the fingers or toes, and stinging or throbbing pain upon warming. Raynaud's phenomenon or disease causes intermittent symptoms, usually lasting minutes, but not permanent symptoms. The red median digits that sometimes develop with carpal tunnel syndrome are chronic, not intermittent or related to cold exposure such as occurs with Raynaud's.

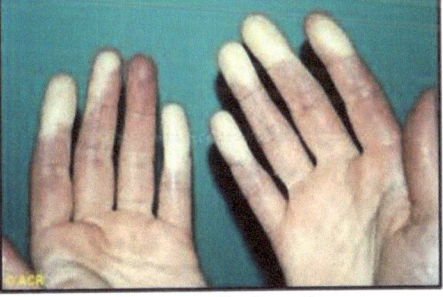

Raynaud's hands

Thenar hypoplasia

There is a syndrome of thenar hypoplasia with X-ray evidence of malformed, underdeveloped thumb phalanges. This can mimic the physical findings of severe carpal tunnel syndrome with thenar atrophy.

Chapter 3 Clinical Exam

Neurologic exam

The physician approaching a patient with numbness, pain, and weakness of the hands should consider a differential diagnosis of: cervical radiculopathy from a disc, syringomyelia, spinal cord disease, Parsonage Turner syndrome causing brachial plexopathy, cerebral disease like a stroke, TIA, or attack of multiple sclerosis, migraine with aura hand sensory symptoms, Pancoast tumor or neurilemoma involving the median cord of the brachial plexus, and entrapment of the median nerve in the carpal tunnel. Numbness of all 5 digits not uncommonly results from median neuropathy at the wrist with carpal tunnel syndrome.

A complete adult neurologic exam should be performed with emphasis on the arms and hands. Deep tendon reflexes in the arms should be normal. Knee and ankle jerks should be normal to rule out generalized polyneuropathy. Muscle bulk of the shoulder, upper arm, forearm, and hand region should be analyzed for atrophy. Complete upper arm muscle testing should be carried out, with especial attention to the strength of flexor pollicis longus, oppenens pollicis, the interossei, and abductor pollicis brevis muscles. Radial pulse and blood pressure should be checked. Sensory exam should include light touch with cotton, sharp/dull discrimination with a pin, vibration with a tuning fork, and 2-point discrimination over the fingertips.

Provocative tests: The Tinel sign

The Tinel sign, tested by tapping the median nerve with the examiner's finger at the wrist over the carpal tunnel and the ulnar nerve at the elbow and inquiring if the patient felt a tingling or electric feeling after the tapping, should be tested. Tinel described his tap test after examining many peripheral nerve injuries. The test may be positive in half of normal persons but may be helpful in analyzing patients with carpal tunnel syndrome, where often times, tapping may bring the patient off the examination table, indicating to the doctor sensitivity of the nerve at just that spot. Like a short in the wire supplying an electric light, movement of the wire at a certain point back and forth may localize the short so that the light flickers on and off. So, likewise a positive Tinel sign at the wrist should indicate irritability of the median at the spot where it was tapped.

My experience is that the sign may be lost as the median nerve is progressively damaged with time and a patient with thenar atrophy and anaesthesia for pin perception over median innervated digits often doesn't have a positive Tinel sign. Tinel's test has a sensitivity (the ability of a test to correctly identify those with the disease) of 48-73% and a specificity (the proportion of patients without disease who test negative) of 30-94%.

There are detractors from this position of helpfulness of the sign, however. Jules Tinel described that tapping the proximal stump of an injured nerve may produce an itching or tingling sensation (fourmillement) in its cutaneous distribution. He concluded that this indicated axonal regeneration. He never mentioned using the sign for entrapment neuropathies, although many standard neurology textbooks state that it is of value in diagnosing CTS. Also, most writers point to Phalen's work as he found Tinel's sign in 73% of 621 hands with alleged CTS, but none of his patients had EMG confirmation and only 40% of his patients had median nerve decompression. The others improved with conservative treatment. Since it is unusual for 60% of hands with CTS to recover without decompression, there is some uncertainty about how many of Phalen's patients actually had CTS. Other writers have found a positive median Tinel sign in the absence of CTS. A study using common CTS clinical features and EMG found a positive Tinel sign in 23/51 or 45% of patients with CTS and a positive Tinel sign in 15/52 or 29% of patients without CTS. These authors concluded that Tinel's sign is of no diagnostic value.

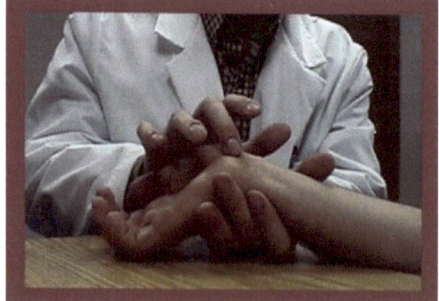

The Tinel Sign
Provocative tests: The Phalen maneuver
To perform the Phalen maneuver the patient should be advised to tell the doctor when the fingers or hand tingles or goes to sleep after dorsiflexing the hands and pressing them together for a minute. Phalen maneuver has a sensitivity of 67-83% and a

specificity of 40-98%. Gelberman, et al, wrote in the *Journal of Bone and Joint Surgery* (Am) in 1981 on "The carpal tunnel syndrome. A study of carpal canal pressures." The authors used a wick catheter inserted through the wrist in 15 persons with CTS and in 12 control subjects. The mean pressure in the carpal canal was elevated significantly in patients with CTS. In patients with CTS the mean pressure was 32 mmHg with the wrist in a neutral position. Ninety degrees of wrist extension increased the mean pressure to 110 mmHg. Control subjects registered 2.5 mgHg with the wrist in neutral position and with extension, the pressure rose to 31 mmHg. Carpal tunnel release produced immediate and sustained reduction in pressure.

These findings indicate that carpal tunnel syndrome results from increased pressure within the tunnel leading to vascular ischemia of the median nerve. Factors that reduce the tunnel size cause the pressure increase. These facts set the stage for understanding how the "nerve goes to sleep" with either flexion or extension positions or how maintenance of a neutral straight-out position decreases the pressure on the nerve. This explains how the neutral carpal tunnel splint may help to treat the syndrome, a treatment modality discussed more thoroughly in Chapter 8.

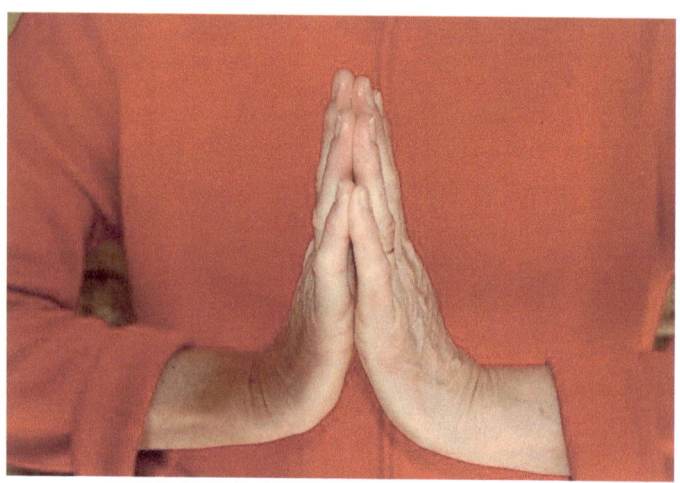

The Phalen Maneuver

Chapter 4 Causes

<u>Associated Medical Conditions</u>
An American trial lawyer will say it's his client, the poor, overworked secretary who types all day that gets carpal tunnel syndrome and that typing, or computer use causes the syndrome. Some persons who type a lot will develop the syndrome, but many others type a lot and never have a problem, so there must be more to it than typing. One study found that among 257 of 314 employees 184 or 70% reported no CTS symptomatology. Of the remaining 76, 70 were interviewed and 10 % met clinical criteria for CTS confirmed by nerve conduction studies in 3.5%. These percentages are comparable to those of the general population risk for CTS. One author felt that milder initial impairment, bilateral baseline symptoms, and positive Phalen sign predicted a poor prognosis.

<u>CTS and computer users</u>
Stevens, et al, wrote a brief communication in *Neurology* in 2000 on "The frequency of carpal tunnel syndrome in computer users at a medical facility." Stevens, et al, stated:

A survey was done of employees who were identified as frequent computer users. Although 29.6% of the employees reported hand paresthesias, only 27 employees (10.5%) met clinical criteria for carpal tunnel syndrome, and in 9 (3.5%) the syndrome was confirmed by nerve conduction studies. Affected and unaffected employees had similar occupations, years using a computer, and time using the computer during the day. The frequency of carpal tunnel syndrome in computer users is similar to that in the general population.

Andersen, et al, wrote in the *JAMA* in 2003 on "Computer Use and Carpal Tunnel syndrome." The authors reported on questionnaires conducted in 2000 and 2001 at 3500 workplaces in Denmark studying the contribution of use of mouse devices and keyboards to the risk of possible CTS with 1 year follow up. The authors studied 9480 persons and reached the conclusion that:

> The occurrence of possible CTS in the right hand was low. The study emphasizes that computer use does not pose a severe occupational hazard for developing symptoms of CTS."

Mediouni, et al, wrote in *J Occup Environ Med* in 2014 on "Is carpal tunnel syndrome related to computer exposure at work? A review and meta-analysis." The authors studied published articles from four databases: PubMed, Embase, Web of Science, and base de Donnees de Sante Publique, and found six studies that met their criteria for inclusion. Their conclusion was: "It was not possible to show an association between computer use and CTS, although some particular work circumstances may be associated with CTS."

Economic burden

The burden here is the cost of providing medical care and lost labor income due to time off.

The economic cost of carpal tunnel syndrome is significant and a study in 1995 estimated approximately 500,000 carpal tunnel decompressions were undertaken every year with an economic cost of $2 billion dollars.

Foley, et al, wrote in the *Am J Ind Med* in 2007 on "The economic burden of carpal tunnel syndrome: long-term earnings of CTS claimants in Washington State." The authors stated.

CTS claimants recover to about half of their pre-injury earnings level relative to that of comparison groups after 6 years; they also endured periods on time-loss three times longer than claimants with upper extremity fractures. CTS surgery claimants had better outcomes than those who did not have surgery.

Cumulative excess loss of earnings of the 4,443 CTS claimants was 197 million dollars to 382 million dollars over 6 years, a loss of 45,000-89,000 dollars per claimant.

CDC guidelines state:

Carpal tunnel syndrome may affect as many as 1.9 million people, and 300,000 to 500,000 surgeries are performed each year to correct this condition.

The Bureau of Labor Statistics reported 26,794 CTS cases involving days from work in 2001, representing a median of 25 days away from work compared with 6 days for all nonfatal injury and illness cases. Most cases involved workers who were aged 25-54 (84%), female and white, non-Hispanic (75%).

Incidence/prevalence rates

The lifetime risk of symptoms of CTS in a specific person is nearly 10%. It's accepted that women have 3 to 4 times the incidence of carpal tunnel syndrome than men do and that women also have small carpal tunnels. The syndrome occurs mostly in adults and is rare in teenagers or children. Commonly persons in their 70's or 80's with CTS have severe median nerve demyelinating neuropathy with thumb base atrophy and fingertip sensory loss for pin, indicating the process has been going on for a long time.

CTS is present in 3.8% of the general population and 1 of every 5 persons with symptoms of pain, numbness, and tingling in the hands is suspect for median neuropathy at the wrist. The incidence rate is 276/100,000 per year with a prevalence rate in women of 9.2% and 6% in men. It occurs bilaterally commonly between the ages of 40-60 years old. Diabetic patients have a prevalence rate of 14% without diabetic neuropathy and 30% with neuropathy. CTS accounted for 0.2% of all U.S. ambulatory care visits in 2006.

Combination of factors

Usually, the syndrome results due to a combination of factors—a congenitally small carpal tunnel by birth, incidental swelling of the wrist due to sprain, trauma, or wrist fracture, diabetes, fluid retention, hypothyroidism, obesity, pregnancy, mechanical problems in the wrist joint, work stress with repeated flexion/extension movement, use of vibrating hand tools, or the development of a cyst or tumor in the tunnel.

Stevens, et al, writing in *Neurology* in 2002 stated:

> The association of occupation and repetitive motion with CTS is controversial. Occupations that require strenuous effort with high repetition, flexed or extended positions of the wrist, and use of vibrating tools seem to be related.

Associated Activities

Understanding that most likely the syndrome develops in the hands of persons with small or compromised carpal tunnels, the following is a discussion of activities that have been associated with carpal tunnel syndrome:

> Persons who have high force, high repetitive manual movements— fix it men, cooks, cashiers, typists, 10 key operators, mouse users, assemblers, bookkeepers, welders and cutters, janitors and cleaners, bank tellers, data processors, construction workers, loggers, dentists.
>
> It occurs in musicians (guitarists, pianists, and violinists), athletes (tennis players, gymnasts,

weightlifters, baseball players, bicyclers, tendon rupture from sports injuries, acute CTS from wrist fracture, nonspecific tenosynovitis), motorcycle riders, seamstresses, barbers, hair stylists, butchers, house cleaners, and gardeners.

It can come from direct wrist trauma.

Meat, poultry, or fish packers, frozen food factory workers, assembly workers, persons who use power tools or vibrating electrical equipment, and jack hammer operators have very high rates of carpal tunnel syndrome.

The symptoms may be set off by a weekend of painting the garage, working in the yard, or writing letters.

CTS occurs seasonally as people use their hands—women at Christmas wrapping presents and writing Christmas cards, students, cramming for final exams in January or May, accountants at April 15th, business employees who input data or manually write end of the month, end of the quarter, or end of the year reports.

Hobbies—persons who sew, knit, crochet, work in the garden, do needlepoint, woodworking, rowing, cooking, painting, drawing, bowling, writing, archery, fly fishing, carpentry, or play video games

Medical conditions

Physiologic—pregnancy, menopause, oral contraceptives, previous ovariectomy, square shaped wrist, short stature

Endocrine—diabetes, acromegaly, hypothyroidism

Anatomic—persistent median artery, thickened transverse ligament, abnormal muscle bellies.

Rheumatological—gout, rheumatoid arthritis, osteoarthritis, systemic lupus erythematosus, scleroderma, sarcoidosis, dermatomyositis, polymyalgia rheumatica

Traumatic—distal radial (Colles) fracture, carpal (lunate) fracture or dislocation

Neoplastic—ganglion, lipoma, cyst, hemangioma, neuroma, Paget's disease, giant cell tumor of flexor sheath, synovial angioma

Hematological—leukemia, multiple myeloma, hemophilia, amyloidosis, bleeding, eosinophilic fasciitis, dyscrasia with hemorrhage in the wrist

Social—alcoholism, obesity

Infectious tuberculosis

Dietary—vitamin deficiency

Other—congestive heart failure, renal failure, arteriovenous shunts for dialysis, lipofibroma or an arborizing lipoma of the median nerve, digital gigantism, median artery thrombosis, Dupytrens contracture, prolonged wrist flexion with decorticate posturing.

CTS during pregnancy

The prevalence of CTS in pregnancy has a wide skew of incidence with authors reporting 0.8% to 70%. This likely reflects different techniques of defining the syndrome. In general CTS during pregnancy is less severe than idiopathic CTS and has a better likelihood of spontaneous resolution. CTS surgery is rarer in women with onset in pregnancy than idiopathic CTS. Pregnant patients with CTS have a probability of improvement which is 3-4 times greater and longer lasting than women with idiopathic CTS. CTS symptoms persist at one year in 50% of patients and in 30% after 3 years. Half of affected women will have tolerable symptoms and 85% will not require further treatment 3 years after delivery. CTS in pregnancy is likely due to fluid retention, hormonal fluctuations, nerve hypersensitivity, and glucose fluctuation levels. The normal diuresis after pregnancy relieves the fluid and also carpal tunnel symptoms.

CTS rarely predicts underlying disease.

Although many medical conditions may be associated with CTS, starting with 386 patients with a diagnosis of CTS and screening for medical diseases such as diabetes, hypothyroidism, or autoimmune disorders resulted in only 2 with diabetes and 2 who were hypothyroid.

Chapter 5 History

Sir James Paget in 1854 first described, but did not name, the symptoms from a compressed median nerve at the wrist. His first patient was a man who developed pain and impaired sensation in the hand from the trauma of a cord drawn tightly around his wrist. In a second case, a tardy median nerve palsy was a consequence of a distal radius fracture; this patient improved with wrist immobilization and thus was also the first description of treatment with a neutral wrist splint, a method still in use today.

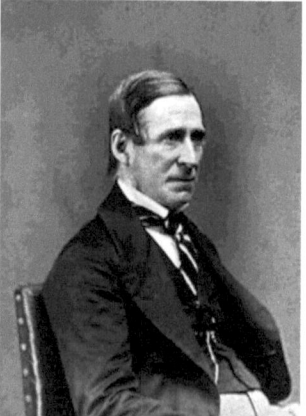

Sir James Pagett

J.J. Putnam described a case of chronic carpal tunnel syndrome in 1880 with purely sensory symptoms occurring mainly at night which he thought was due to "the smaller branches or terminal filaments of the sensitive nerves supplying the affected districts." The condition was called "Putnam acroparesthesia." Putnam described:

...disturbances of a subjective sensibility of the skin, giving rise to what is popularly known as numbness recurring periodically, coming on especially at night...in some cases simply letting the arm hang out of the bed or shaking it about for some moments would drive the numbness away.

J.J. Putnam

Ramsey Hunt wrote three reports of thenar atrophy with no sensory symptoms between the years 1909 through 1914. He thought that the problem related to compression of the thenar branch of the median nerve at the wrist. Hunt introduced the terms "Occupational neuritis" and "neural atrophy of the hand."

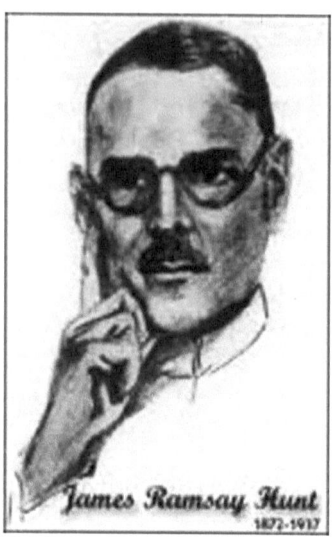

Ramsay Hunt

Marie and Foix writing in 1913 gave the first comprehensive clinical and pathological assessment of a non-traumatic median nerve lesion at the wrist. They reported to the French Neurological Society a case of an 80-year-old man with bilateral thenar eminence atrophy. Marie and Foix's case is described below.

> The nerves appeared normal with exception of the median nerve. The median nerve starting in the distal forearm shows a slow increase in volume. Immediately proximal to the annular ligament a nodular thickening is present which looks and feels like a neuroma. Underlying the annular ligament, however, the nerve suddenly becomes thin…An enormous increase in the connective tissue (was seen)

interfascicular as well as intrafascicular. The myelin sheets are progressively diminished from the beginning of the nodular thickening and at the constriction they are nearly completely absent.

An important comment in the same article stating that "transection of the ligament could stop the development of these phenomena" was neglected for decades.

H. Galloway in 1924 performed the first recorded carpal tunnel release surgery. In a letter written in 1925 he described a woman with clinical signs and symptoms of CTS who experienced improved sensation of her index finger following surgical exploration of the median nerve at the wrist. Portions of Galloway's letter follows:

There was marked wasting of the thenar eminence and trophic changes in the nails of the index finger and thumb. On 11 March 1924 the condition of the median nerve was explored from the flexor crease at the wrist downward for an inch and upward for 2 inches. Its appearance was entirely normal. Following this operation there was some improvement in sensation in the index finger.

Sir James Learmonth described the first surgical release of the transverse carpal ligament for median nerve neuropathy in 1933 in *Surgical Clin North Am* in an article entitled "The principle of decompression in the treatment of certain diseases of peripheral nerves."

Moersch, neurologist at the Mayo Clinic, wrote in 1938 in an article entitled "Median thenar neuritis." He revived the idea of Marie and Foix that the location of the lesion was in the wrist. In the early nineteenth century the literature had been confused with thoracic outlet syndrome and involvement of the seventh cervical root by a cervical rib. The failure of cervical rib removal to relieve the symptoms led investigators to reconsider a location of the problem at the median wrist. Moersch said:

> The explanation for the development of this specific form of median neuritis is probably on an anatomic basis…is likely that the thenar branch…is compressed either by direct trauma or by continued irritation…Sensory disturbances probably are attributable to an involvement of the main trunk of the median nerve at the annular ligament.

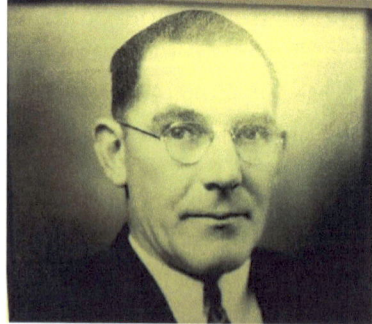

F.P. Moersch

Brain, Wright, and Wilkinson first reported surgical treatment of 6 cases of carpal tunnel syndrome in 1947.

George Phalen's publications, starting in 1950 were important in spreading general knowledge regarding median neuropathy at the wrist. He and his associates gave it the name "carpal tunnel syndrome." He confirmed the performance of the Phalen maneuver and Tinel sign as helpful clinical diagnostic tests. Phalen wrote:

Tinel's sign over the median nerve at the wrist was elicited in every case. This is a tingling sensation, radiating out into the hand, which is obtained by light percussion over the median nerve at the wrist.

Although pressure within the carpal tunnel is increased by extension of the wrist, the numbness and paresthesias in the fingers of these patients could be increased by sharply flexing the wrist for a period of 60 seconds. Prompt improvement in these symptoms would result with release of the wrist from the flexed position.

We examined 71 patients with spontaneous compression of the median nerve in the carpal tunnel...The patient's symptoms of pain and paresthesias in the median nerve distribution may be readily relieved by sectioning the transverse carpal ligament to decompress the median nerve in the carpal tunnel.

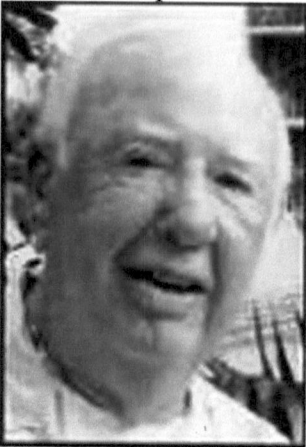

George Phalen

Chapter 6 EMG Diagnosis

History

Early Greek physicians used electrical eels to shock "ailments" out of the bodies of their patients. Swammerdam (1637-1680) discovered that stroking the nerve to the gastrocnemius of a frog produced a contraction. He also probably used electrical stimulation experiments 134 years before Galvanni. Redi (1626-1698) first discovered in 1666 a specialized muscle of the electric ray fish (the electric eel) which generated electricity. In 1792 Galvanni wrote in *De Viribus Elecriticitatis in Motu Musclari Commentarius* that electricity could initiate muscle contraction. The first electrical stimulation of a human nerve is usually ascribed to Galvani's nephew, Giovanni Aldini (1762-1834) in 1804. However, a letter in the June 2014 journal of *Muscle & Nerve* reported that "Johann Christian Reil (1759-1812), professor for therapy at the University of Halle, described electrical nerve stimulation in himself in 1792."

The action potential was described by De Bois Reymond and Bernstein in 1865. Duchenne, Matteucci, and Sarlandier used intramuscular needles in their studies. In 1852 Helmolz first measured nerve conduction velocities in humans. Marey in 1890 recorded muscle contraction activity and introduced the term "electromyography."

In 1922 Gasser and Erlanger used an oscilloscope to display the electrical activity in muscles. Hodes, et al, in 1948 demonstrated the first electrophysiological evidence of abnormality of human peripheral nerve disease by showing slowing of conduction velocity in injured regenerating nerve. The invention of high-grade electrical equipment during World War II accelerated the development of the science. Dawson and Scott in 1949 showed a means of averaging sensory nerves by using superimposed photographic pictures of nerve potentials and suggested that the technique could be used to study nerve disease. In 1956 Simpson reported prolonged median motor distal latency across the carpal tunnel in CTS. Thomas and Lambert confirmed their results in 1962. In 1958 Gilliat and Sears reported slow median sensory nerve conduction across the carpal tunnel in patients with CTS.

Since these early studies clinical research efforts have refined electromyography techniques to make them more specific and reliable for diagnosis. The American Association of Electrodiagnositic Medicine has helped educate physicians and technicians trained in EMG technology and published a number of articles on the EMG diagnosis of carpal tunnel syndrome and other articles on neuromuscular disease. EMG is the gold standard for evaluating carpal tunnel syndrome, yet one study found that 21% of patients who had carpal tunnel surgery did not have a preoperative EMG study.

Electromyographic studies (EDX) consist of nerve conduction studies and a needle exam. The physician takes a history and performs a neurologic exam before the study is performed. Patients are informed to avoid creams and lotions on their arms or legs before coming to the lab. The test usually takes 1 to 2 hours and is mildly uncomfortable. Temperature of the limbs should be determined and then heated up by a hair dryer or inserting the limb in warm water for 10 minutes. Every lab should establish their own temperature controlled normal values for amplitude, latency, and conduction velocity for the various nerves or else use published normal values.

An assessment of a patient with numbness and tingling, pain, or weakness in one or both arms should be considered as having an EMG problem located at the nerve root, brachial plexus, or along the branch of a specific peripheral nerve. Commonly the examiner will perform median and ulnar palmar sensory and radial sensory studies along with median and ulnar motor conduction studies. The sensory studies usually analyze the latency and amplitude of evoked nerves, comparing the results with normal, while the motor studies consist of latency, amplitude, and conduction velocity measurements. Often times F waves of the median and ulnar nerves are obtained which studies the segment of the individual nerves at the root level. Comparison with median or ulnar motor and sensory limbs in the contralateral limb gives perspective regarding slowing or normality of the various nerve fibers.

Needle exam of at least 5 muscles in the symptomatic limb should be performed choosing muscles representing the nerves of the brachial plexus that go into the arm. This would mean sampling muscles innervated by C5 through T1.

Palmar median and ulnar sensory studies, stimulating at the palm and recording 8 cm proximally give the highest return for analysis of carpal tunnel syndrome. Many labs also do orthodromic or antidromic median and ulnar sensory studies. Still 10-15% of patients with a clinical diagnosis of CTS will have normal NCSs, reflecting a sensitivity of 85-90%.

Literature Review

P.K. Thomas in an article entitled "Motor nerve conduction in the carpal tunnel" published in *Neurology* in 1960 a report on median motor conduction velocities and distal motor latencies in a group of normal controls and in patients with carpal tunnel syndrome. Concentric needle exam of the abductor pollicis brevis muscle was also performed, but this was normal in all patients. Normal distal motor latencies were mostly less than 4.5 msec and affected clinically suspected CTS patients ranged from 3 to 13 msec. Two patients had very long latencies of 19.5 and 26 msec and in 6 patients the median nerve was totally inexcitable. The most frequent latencies were over 4.5 msec. No sensory latencies were performed. Thomas reported "...the latency of the muscle action potential in the abductor pollicis brevis was abnormally prolonged in approximately two-thirds." Median conduction velocity was also moderately reduced over the forearm and upper arm in patients with a delay at the wrist.

In 1967 Thomas, et al, from the Mayo Clinic reported in 1967 in the *Archives of Neurology* on "Electrodiagnostic Aspects of the Carpal Tunnel Syndrome." This report consisted of "all consecutive cases seen at the Mayo Clinic between 1956 and 1963 in which there was 1) a final diagnosis of carpal tunnel syndrome, 2) an electromyographic examination, and 3) surgical decompression of the median nerve."

Thomas, et al, reported on a total of 300 patients 70 men and 230 women. All patients had median and ulnar conduction velocity and distal motor latency assessment. Needle exam of muscles of the forearm and hand was performed in 213 patients and two thirds of the patients had median sensory studies. Patient average age was 52 years old (18-84) and in over half (176) CTS affected both hands. Eighty-one patients had only the right hand involved and 43 patients had only the left hand involved. Normal conduction velocity of the median motor fibers between elbow and wrist ranged from 49 to 74 m/sec with a mean of 59 m/sec. CTS patients had a mean of conduction velocity of 53 m/sec which is 6 m/sec below the mean for normal.

At the Mayo EMG lab median distal motor latency values ranged from 2.5 to 4.7 msec. CTS patients had prolongation of distal latency more than 4.7 msec in 286 hands (60%); failure to detect and a thenar action potential in 21 hands (4.4%), and a difference in distal latency between the symptomatic and asymptomatic hand of more than 1 msec, even though both values were within normal limits in 13 hands (2.7%). Prolonged distal median motor latencies went up to as high as 14.4 msec in symptomatic hands.

All patients had normal ulnar motor conduction velocities and distal motor latencies. Orthodromic median sensory studies were performed by stimulating the index finger and recording at the wrist. Normal values at the Mayo lab for median sensory responses varied from 2.1 to 3.5 msec with a mean of 2.8 msec. Abnormalities of the median sensory fibers were found in 85% of patients and consisted of prolongation of latency beyond 3.5 msec in 120 hands, failure to get a response in 174 patients (50%), and a difference in latency between symptomatic and the asymptomatic hand of more than 0.5 msec even though both values were within normal limits in one patient.

Needle exam results of the abductor pollicis brevis and opponens pollicis muscles were performed in 213 patients. Fibrillation potentials were found in 95 patients (44%). In 17 patients fasciculation potentials were also seen while 8 cases had only fasciculation potentials but no fibrillation potentials. No patient with normal sensory study had fibrillation potentials on needle exam. Thomas, et al, summarized their findings:

> Some patients with symptoms of CTS in both hands had EMG abnormalities only on the clinically more severe side.

> Some patients with unilateral symptoms had EMG findings bilaterally.

Patients with symptoms for only a short time had abnormalities on motor nerve studies less often than those with symptoms of longer duration.

Recovery after surgical decompression of the median nerve was generally excellent; 81 % reported good results from surgery (100% or 75% improved), 10% reported fair results (50% or 25% improved), and 9% had poor results (condition unchanged or worse).

EMG findings provided no clue to postoperative prognosis.

Conduction abnormalities on EMG can be evident within days after onset of symptoms but are more likely when symptoms have been present for a long time.

Needle exam is not as helpful in CTS as studies of nerve conduction.

EMG abnormalities may be found among patients with CTS who have no neurologic deficit, but in the presence of marked neurologic impairment, the EMG is always abnormal.

This landmark article is still very relevant today and full of useful information.

In 1984 Evans and Daube wrote on "A Comparison of Three Electrodiagnostic Methods of Diagnosing Carpal Tunnel Syndrome," in *Muscle &*

Nerve. The authors compared residual latency, terminal latency index, and median and ulnar palm-wrist sensory latency for 140 hands of 88 consecutive patients referred to the EMG lab with a clinical impression of possible carpal tunnel syndrome but who had no clinical or electrodiagnostic evidence of other disease. Fifty-one percent of the patients had an abnormal median distal motor latency. Sixty-four percent of those in whom palmar studies were done had abnormal median palm-wrist sensory latencies. In hands with normal motor distal latency (68), palmar stimulation studies were abnormal in 59%. None of the 10 median neuropathies identified only by an abnormal difference between median and ulnar palmar-wrist latencies had abnormal residual latency or terminal latency index. The authors concluded that: "median sensory latency and the latency difference between median and ulnar sensory nerve at the same distance across the carpal tunnel comprise the most sensitive test for CTS."

Monga, Shanks, and Poole writing in the *Archives of Physical Medicine and Rehabilitaion* in 1985 on "Sensory Palmar Stimulation in the Diagnosis of Carpal Tunnel Syndrome," concluded that "the use of measurement of median palmar sensory latency under the flexor retinaculum adds to the sensitivity of the nerve conduction studies in the diagnosis of CTS."

Stevens wrote AAEE minimonograph #26: The Electrodiagnosis of Carpal Tunnel Syndrome in 1987 published in *Muscle & Nerve* and he updated the same paper again in 1997 . Stevens reported:

The Mayo Clinic EMG lab studied residents of Rochester, Minnesota through the years 1961 through 1980. The study had 1016 patients with a clinical diagnosis of carpal tunnel syndrome and 505 (885 hands) had EMG studies—NCV and needle exams. The EMG was positive in in 73% of affective hands which was a community study rather than patients selected in a surgical or EMG laboratory based series.

In the Rochester study 37.5% of 829 hands had prolonged (>4.6msec) median motor nerve distal latencies and 1.9% had no response.

When less than 4.7 msec the median motor nerve distal latency should be compared with the ulnar motor nerve distal latency and if the median value is 1.8 msec longer than the ulnar, the median can be considered abnormal. Using this comparison, the number of abnormal median nerve distal latencies increased to 50%.

The median motor distal latency can be considered abnormal on the symptomatic side when it is greater than or equal to 1.0 msec longer than the median motor latency on the opposite side. Using this criterion only 6 hands not already abnormal were found to be abnormal. Since CTS is bilateral in 55% of patients, this comparison is rarely helpful.

Very rarely median motor distal latencies are abnormal when sensory nerve latencies are normal. This is likely due to more extensive compression of fascicles containing motor fibers or due to frequent exit of the motor branch through a separate opening in the carpal ligament where it may be compressed. This is rare and only happened in 10 hands in the Rochester study and in 3.9% of hands in another large series. In the Rochester study 202 hands studied with palmar sensory stimulation had no abnormal prolonged motor latency.

In the Rochester study the CMAP (compound muscle action potential) was abnormal (<4 mV or no response) in 15.4%, a finding representing advanced carpal tunnel syndrome and an indication for surgery.

Repetitive firing of motor nerve fibers in CTS was first noted by Simpson in 1956 and rarely occurs as a short buzz of small potentials after stimulation.

The Rochester study had slowing of conduction velocity in the forearm in 86 (11%) associated with prolongation of the distal motor nerve latency. Fibers that innervate the lumbricals lie more posteriorly in the carpal tunnel than those innervating thenar muscles, so the lumbrical motor fibers are protected from compression against the flexor retinaculm. Therefore, lumbrical sparing may occur in CTS and recording from the 2nd lumbrical and comparing the median and ulnar motor latencies is a technique that improves the sensitivity of motor nerve conduction studies. The second lumbrical motor point is recorded and the median and ulnar nerves are stimulated at the same distance at the wrist. A >0.4 msec difference between the median and ulnar latencies is significant. This technique is also helpful in patients with severe carpal tunnel syndrome in whom there is no median response at the wrist while recording from the abductor pollicis brevis because a lumbrical response may be obtained in this situation.

Martin-Gruber median-ulnar nerve communications are found in 15-30% of normal persons which is inherited as an autosomal dominant trait and is bilateral in 68%. This occurs when axons leave the main trunk of the median nerve or the anterior interosseous nerve and "cross over" to the main trunk of the ulnar nerve, providing a pathway to the thenar muscles that bypasses the carpal tunnel. This may be noted by finding, with ulnar motor nerve stimulation, the amplitude is lower during proximal stimulation, whereas with median nerve stimulation, it is higher during proximal stimulation. Another clue here is with ulnar motor stimulation, there will be an initial positive dip in thenar CMAP at the elbow that is not seen at the wrist.

Prolongation or absence of the distal sensory latency has been reported in 53-98% of cases. In the Rochester study, the median sensory nerve latencies were prolonged (>3.5 msec) or absent in 64%.

To exclude a peripheral neuropathy as the cause of prolonged median nerve latencies, the ulnar motor and sensory conduction studies should be a routine part of the examination. If ulnar neuropathy is found, the median sensory latencies should be compared with the superficial radial sensory nerve because entrapment of this nerve is rare.

Starting in the 1970's an improvement in diagnostic accuracy occurred using latency measurement over shorter segments from palm to wrist. It is now known that palmar stimulation is more sensitive than orthodromic or antidromic stimulation for diagnosing carpal tunnel syndrome. The median and ulnar nerves are stimulated in the midpalm 8 cm distal to recording electrodes over the wrist. Normally the ulnar and median sensory latencies do not differ by more than 0.2 msec.

In the Rochester study, median palmar sensory distal latencies were abnormal in 91% of affected right hands and in 82% of affected left hands, with an overall positivity of 87%. The SNAP (sensory nerve action potential) was reduced by 44%.

Sometimes the antidromic radial sensory nerve may be studied, usually by stimulating the radial sensory nerve in the dorsal forearm 10 cm above a recording electrode over the dorsal proximal phalanx of the thumb. The radial nerve is generally less affected by neuropathy and comparison of median/radial sensory latencies may be helpful using <0.5 msec as a normal difference between the two.

When NCS are abnormal in one limb or when the patient's symptoms are bilateral, ulnar, and median sensory NCSs should be done on the opposite side. If they are normal, then no further NCSs are needed. If CTS is found on the opposite side, a median motor NCS should be considered, especially if the opposite hand sensory study is very abnormal. If the symptomatic hand has normal NCSs, there is no need to perform NCSs on the opposite asymptomatic hand.

The needle examination is also important and muscles need to be sampled to rule in or out a cervical radiculopathy or carpal tunnel syndrome. One study found that in 104 patients with surgically proven cervical radiculopathy, 18 patients also had carpal tunnel syndrome. This suggests that CTS and cervical radiculopathy can coexist in the same patient.

The needle exam, especially of thenar muscles was the least sensitive part of the EMG exam. Also the needle exam of the base of the thumb hurts and is painful. Buchthal et al found reduced recruitment and prolonged duration in 50 % of muscles, polyphasic potentials in 60%, and spontaneous activity in 50%. Fasciculations were found in 18% of muscles.

In the Rochester community study, needle exam of the abductor pollicis brevis muscle was normal in 59% and 41% had decreased recruitment or motor unit potential abnormalities. Fibrillation with or without positive waves was seen in 18%. Thomas et al, studying a more severely affected group of patients found fibrillation potentials in 44%.

Occasionally spontaneously discharging motor unit potentials are found in the thenar muscles of patients with CTS. These discharges may look like single, very regularly firing potentials or as doublets or triplets in a pattern like myokymia.

EMG data may be used to give an indication for operation, although this is mainly a clinical decision. Factors such as the age and general health of the patient and the severity of symptoms should be considered. Patients with mild disease or the pregnant patient may get by with wrist splinting or local steroid injection. CTS symptoms are not always progressive and sometimes resolve spontaneously. Sensory loss, thenar muscle weakness, and wasting usually warrant more aggressive therapy. In a patient with decreased SNAP and thenar CMAP amplitudes and prolonged median motor and palmar sensory latencies, surgery should be considered.

Pronounced prolongation of motor and sensory nerve latencies may be an indication for operation, but symptoms do not correlate well with latencies. Fibrillation potentials on needle exam and/or decreased recruitment and large motor units are usually associated with more severe median compression and suggest that an operation is necessary.

There is no universally accepted means of grading the severity of CTS, yet a combination of clinical and EMG findings may be helpful. Stevens proposed:

Mild CTS—prolonged (relative or absolute) sensory or mixed NAP distal latency (orthodromic, antidromic, or palmar) +/- SNAP amplitude below the lower limit of normal.

Moderate CTS—abnormal median sensory latencies as above and (relative or absolute) prolongation of median motor distal latency.

Severe CTS—prolonged median motor and sensory distal

latencies, with either an absent SNAP or mixed NAP, or low amplitude or absent thenar CMAP. Needle examination often reveals fibrillations, reduced recruitment, and motor unit potential changes.

In 1993 the American Association of Electrodiagnostic Medicine, American Academy of Neurology, and the American Academy of Physical Medicine and Rehabilitation published in *Muscle & Nerve* a "Practice Parameter for Electrodiagnostic Studies In Carpal Tunnel syndrome: A Summary Statement" involving many members of the above various organization and chaired by Dr. Charles Jablecki. This was a literature review and Medline search of 488 articles and abstracts along with 81 articles on electrodiagnostic studies published between 1986 and 1991 with the key words "carpal tunnel syndrome", "nerve compression", or "wrist injury."

The committee concluded that this literature provides convincing scientific evidence that median and sensory and motor NCS's:

Are valid and reproducible clinical laboratory studies.

Confirm a clinical diagnosis of CTS in patients with a high degree of sensitivity and specificity.

The committee also said that comparison of the sensitivities of the several different median NCS's evaluated demonstrated that:

1. Median sensory NCS's confirm the clinical diagnosis of CTS more often than do median motor NCS's.

2.The median sensory or mixed nerve conduction from wrist to digit (13-14 cm) is less sensitive for confirmation of the clinical diagnosis of CTS compared to:

2a. Techniques which evaluate median sensory or mixed nerve conduction over a short (7-8 cm) conduction distance across the carpal tunnel, e.g. palmar studies.

2b. Techniques which compare sensory or mixed nerve conduction of the median nerve through the carpal tunnel to sensory or mixed nerve conduction of the ulnar nerve in the same hand.

In 2002 the same organizations as above published in *Muscle & Nerve* "Practice parameter: electrodiagnostic studies in carpal tunnel syndrome." This article included an additional 113 articles for review. The committee's recommendations were "identical to those made and endorsed in 1993" …"with the clarification of recommendation 1 and 2a and the addition of 2c based on new evidence."

1. Perform a median sensory NCS across the wrist with a conduction distance of 13 to 14 cm. If the result is abnormal, comparison of the result of the median sensory NCS

to the result of a sensory NCS of one other adjacent sensory nerve in the symptomatic limb.

2a Comparison of median sensory or mixed nerve conduction across the wrist over a short (7 to 8 cm) conduction distance with ulnar sensory nerve conduction across the wrist over the same short (7 to 8 cm) conduction distance.

2c Comparison of median sensory or mixed nerve conduction through the carpal tunnel to sensory or mixed NCSs of proximal (forearm) or distal (digit) segments of the median nerve in the same limb.

NICE guidelines for management of CTS posted in 2012 stated: "Refer for electromyography and nerve conduction studies if the diagnosis is uncertain."

Chapter 7 X-ray, Ultrasound, MRI Scan

X-ray of the wrist or neck may be performed as part of the work up of carpal tunnel syndrome, particularly if there has been wrist or neck trauma. X-ray of the neck may show vertebral fracture or dislocation, disc space narrowing, or cervical osteoarthritis indicating cervical radiculopathy. X-ray of Colles' fracture, a break in the distal radius above the wrist usually caused by falling forward with the wrist dorsiflexed as it strikes the ground, may by bony encroachment or scarring bind the median nerve in the carpal tunnel.

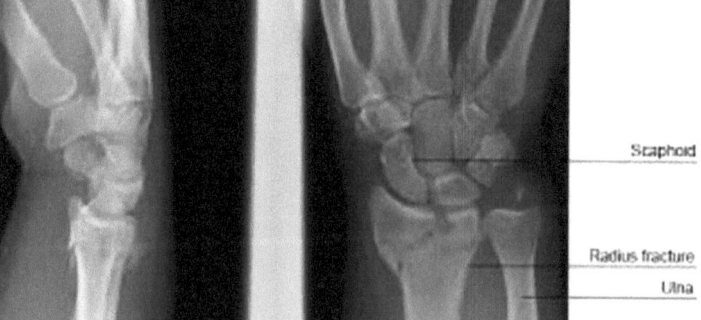

Scaphoid

Radius fracture
Ulna

X-ray Colles' Fracture
Ultrasound

In 2012 the American Association of Neuromuscular & Electrodiagnostic Medicine published in *Muscle & Nerve* "Evidence-Based Guideline: Neuromuscular Ultrasound for The Diagnosis Of Carpal Tunnel Syndrome." This was a multi-authored "Practice Guideline" by an expert panel of physicians specializing in neurology, physical medicine and rehabilitation, and radiology. Neuromuscular ultrasound over the past 20 years has demonstrated focal enlargement of the median nerve at the wrist and abnormalities that would not be appreciated by electrodiagnostic studies such as compressive cysts, tumors, and vessels. The panel asked 2 questions:

1. What is the accuracy of median nerve cross-sectional area enlargement as measured with ultrasound for the diagnosis of CTS?

2. What added value, if any does neuromuscular ultrasound provide over electrodiagnostic studies alone for the diagnosis of CTS?

Literature Review

A systematic review of 240 articles from 1990 through May 2001 was performed, and studies were classified according to the American Academy of Neurology criteria for rating articles of diagnostic accuracy. The results were that neuromuscular ultrasound measurement of median nerve cross-sectional area at the wrist is accurate and may be offered as a diagnostic test for CTS (Level A). The committee also found that neuromuscular ultrasound probably adds value to electrodiagnostic studies when diagnosing CTS and should be considered in screening for structural abnormalities at the wrist in those with CTS (Level B). Bifid median nerves at the wrist were detected in 2-13% of patients with CTS. Persistent median arteries occurred in 9-13% of those with CTS. Also, tenosynovitis in 6% and accessory muscles within the wrist in 3% were found in patients with CTS. Occult ganglia causing median mononeuropathy were seen in 25% of the CTS patients. Rarely seen problems seen on ultrasound were: traumatic neuromas, Schwannomas, lipofibromatous hamartomas, ganglion cysts, thrombosed persistent median arteries, an abcess, and compressive gouty tophus.

The article stressed that screening for structural abnormalities of the wrist which caused CTS was higher in patients with just unilateral CTS, as most patients have bilateral CTS. The authors stressed:

> that neuromuscular ultrasound evaluation of the wrist in those with CTS allows assessment of median nerve cross-sectional area and the presence of structural abnormalities, and this complements well the information obtained during an electrodiagnostic study (which is the gold standard for diagnosis of CTS).

Zyluk, et al, wrote in *Handchir Mikrochir Plast Chir* in 2014 on "Does ultrasonography contribute significantly to the diagnosis of carpal tunnel syndrome?" The objective of this study was to investigate sonographic parameters of the median nerve in patients diagnosed clinically with carpal tunnel syndrome. The authors sonographically studied 185 wrists in 185 patients, 149 (81%) women and 36 (19%) men with the clinical diagnosis of CTS. Cross-sectional area of the median nerve was measured at the forearm and at the carpal tunnel inlet, and also the height of the nerve at the tunnel inlet and in the narrowest site in the carpal tunnel. Severity of the disease was assessed by the Levine questionaire. The authors found no correlation between sonographic data and severity of the syndrome as expressed by the Levine scores. Zyluk, et al, concluded:

> Sonography of the median nerve contributes little to the diagnosis of a clinically relevant carpal tunnel syndrome and its routine use is not justified.

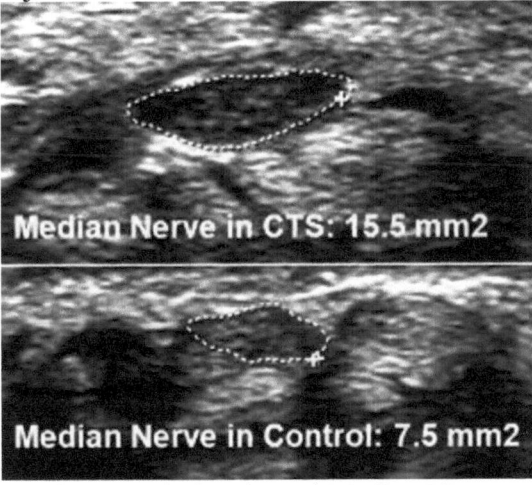

Ultrasound of Enlarged Median Nerve

MRI scan

MRI reports for diagnosis of CTS appeared in the mid-1980s and a number of small sample size studies have been reported. MRI imaging of peripheral nerves is difficult as peripheral nerves on MRI resemble vessels and may appear isotense with muscle. MRI has been used frequently in CTS but its role in routine practice is not established. MRI utility in cases with neoplasm such as neurofibromas, arthritis with gouty tophi, rheumatoid tenosynovitis, and congenital anomalies such as aberrant lumbricals, is valid, but these are not relevant issues in most cases.

Literature Review

Goodman and Gilliatt reported on "The Effect of Treatment On Median Nerve Conduction In Patients With The Carpal Tunnel Syndrome" in 1961 in the *Annals of Physical Medicine*. This was a very early work uniting NCS and surgery on 44 patients (47 hands) with relatively severe clinical and electrophysiological CTS. Thirteen out of thirty-three patients had absent orthodromic median sensory potentials. Three patients had severe, 2 moderate, and 1 mild thenar wasting. Twelve cases had severe (>10 msec) median distal motor latencies, 14 had moderate (7-14 msec) and 15 had moderate (5-6 msec) delay; in 5 patients the distal median motor nerve was inexcitable.

These were a group of patients with chronic CTS. This is what Mr. Valentine Logue, the hand surgeon, reported regarding physical inspection of these nerves:

No abnormality of caliber of the nerve was seen in 13 cases, although in four of these the nerve appeared to be abnormally vascular when the tourniquet was released. Some broadening or flattening of the nerve was seen in five cases, while a

definite constriction under the
retinaculum was seen in three others.
Only two cases showed a marked
swelling proximal to the retinaculum;
in both of them the median nerve was
electrically inexcitable before
operation. In another case, however,
the median nerve was also electrically
inexcitable preoperatively, but no
abnormality was seen on inspection of
the nerve at operation.

One study reported in 2002 by Jarvik, et al, in
Neurology entitled "MR nerve imaging in a
prospective cohort of patients with suspected carpal
tunnel syndrome" studied120 patients with clinically
suspected CTS. The authors reported finding an
increased median nerve signal of 15.8 mm in patients
with suspected CTS versus a signal of 11.8 mm in
normals. The report concluded that the reliability of
MRI is high, but the accuracy is only moderate when
compared with a research-definition reference
standard (NCS).

Schmidt and Visser wrote in *Muscle & Nerve*
in 2008 on "Carpal Tunnel syndrome: Clinical And
Sonographic Follow-up After Surgery." The author's
aims were to study changes in median nerve size at
the proximal carpal tunnel after surgery compared to
conservative treatment and the predictive value of
sonography in relation to the clinical outcome after
surgery. Schmidt and Visser stated that "high-
resolution sonography, with measurement of the
median nerve cross-sectional at the proximal carpal
tunnel inlet, has the same accuracy as

electrophysiological studies for the diagnosis of CTS." Schmidt and Visser reported:

> Sonography at the time of diagnosis was not a predictor of postoperative outcome, but in this study only a relatively small number of patients had a poor postoperative outcome.

Kim, et al, wrote in 2011 in *Muscle & Nerve* on "Carpal Tunnel Syndrome: Clinical, Electrophysiological, And Ultrasonographic Ratio After Surgery." Twenty-four individuals with CTS were evaluated using the Boston questionaire, nerve conduction studies, and ultrasound, preoperatively and at 3 weeks and 3 months postoperatively. Kim, et al, reported:

> Improved symptom scores decreased cross-sectional area (CSA) and decreased cross-sectional area ratio were observed in the first 3 weeks, post-operatively.

> The ratios between the CSA at the sites of enlargement and unaffected areas correlated significantly with the Padua classification, although the coefficient was not superior to the coefficient of CSA at the maximal swelling site.

> Conclusions: Symptoms improved more rapidly than function after surgery. Measurement of the ultrasonographic CSA ratio may

provide clinicians with a useful assessment tool after surgery.

Some MRI studies have found decreased T2 signal in the median nerve in the carpal tunnel which correlates with poor outcome. It is thought that T2 signal decrease of the median nerve reflects fibrosis and amyloid deposition. A recent study by Lindbert, et al, published in 2013 in *European Radiology* on "Diffusion tensor imaging of the median nerve in recurrent carpal tunnel syndrome—initial experience." The authors found "a specific pattern of DTI changes in the median nerve was identified in patients with recurrent CTS." Patients showed reduced apparent diffusion coefficient (ADC), reduced axial diffusivity (AD) and radial diffusivity (RD) along the median nerve compared with controls." These changes were thought to represent endoneural fibrosis and correlated with nerve conduction velocity. The authors thought that that "DTI is a promising technique in recurrent carpal tunnel syndrome."

Oge, et al, writing in *Turkish Neurosurgery* in 2014 on "Quantitative MRI analysis of idiopathic carpal tunnel syndrome "set out to find parametric ratios for the diagnosis and pathology of carpal tunnel syndrome using MRI. They examined 27 female carpal tunnel patients and 21 normal females. They found that the "proportion of the contents of the carpal tunnel is increased in the carpal tunnel patients." They also noted that palmar bowing was increased, and the median nerve cross section area was increased at the proximal entrance of the carpal tunnel. The authors noted that Phalen had postulated that the volume of the contents of the carpal tunnel was increased in CTS patients, an increase that can be demonstrated by MRI imaging.

Summary
Electrodiagnostic studies are the "gold standard" for evaluating carpal tunnel syndrome. CTS is a median neuropathy and best studied by a physiological technique that studies nerve function, i.e. nerve conduction studies. An example of the comparison between an "anatomical" versus a "neurophysiological" test would be a patient with myocardial infarction and cardiac arrest who hasn't regained consciousness in the ICU. A CAT scan of that patient's brain (an anatomical test) may be entirely normal but an EEG (a neurophysiological test of function) may be flat, indicating poor prognosis for the patient.

Ultrasound and MRI scanning are useful additional studies that add anatomical insights to the pathology of what is going on in the carpal tunnel. Suspected tumors or masses may be imaged with these techniques and sometimes provide additional helpful clinical information. Yet, many studies of the median nerves on direct visualization at surgery appeared normal. Patients with repeat CTS due to previous unsuccessful median nerve release and continuing symptoms of carpal tunnel syndrome may benefit from ultrasound or MRI scanning.

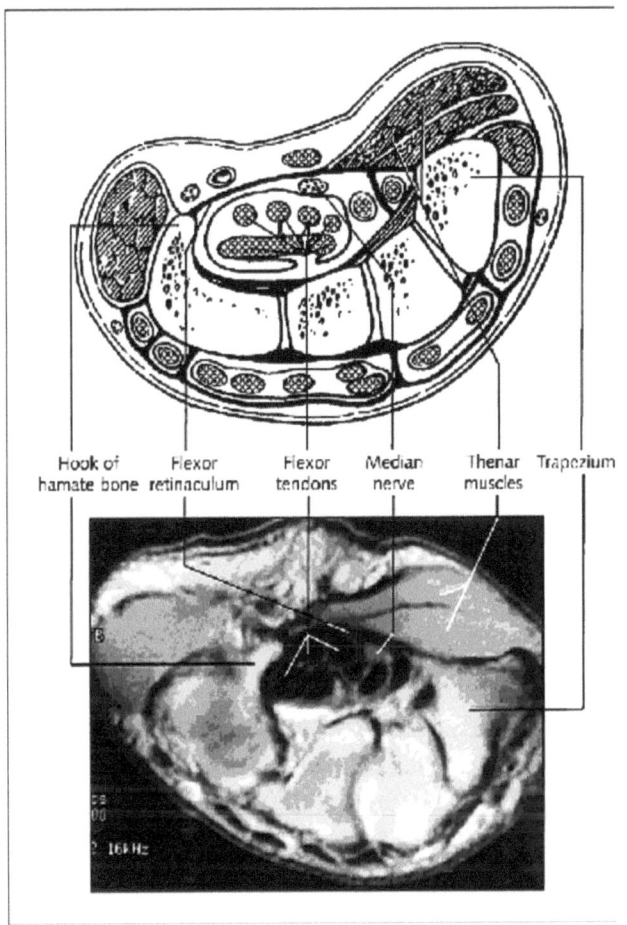

Hook of   Flexor   Flexor   Median   Thenar   Trapezium
hamate bone retinaculum   tendons   nerve   muscles

MRI Scan of The Carpal Tunnel

Chapter 8 Rest, Medication, Splinting

<u>Rest</u>

The first treatment idea is resting the hand. The patient should be encouraged to think about how they use their hands in their daily routine. They should avoid flexion/extension movements or sustained bent postures of the wrist that may aggravate their symptoms. Patients should be advised to rest their wrists and hands from time to time. They should alternate tasks to reduce pressure on their wrists-- delegating tasks and modifying daily activities such as hobbies, cleaning, and work out routines. This idea sounds simple, but it is difficult to do. However, it is very important. Persons who make their living with their hands and also have CTS can't rest their hands well and this makes their treatment more difficult.

I advised one middle aged lady with early carpal tunnel symptoms who had been clipping with garden snips around her roses in the back yard to quit doing the clipping activity and I never heard from her again. Another man got severe painful nighttime hand paresthesiae after several days of stapling a wire fence to a succession of fence posts on his farm over the weekend. I told him he should quit this activity and although he is a chronic patient for another neurologic problem, I never heard about his hands bothering him again.

One study reported the natural history of untreated CTS in 441 affected hands with idiopathic CTS. Twenty-one percent of hands improved over 10-15 months of follow-up without active intervention although 68% of the patients made efforts to reduce occupational and recreational hand stress. Thirty-two percent changed either their hobby or their work. A shorter history, younger age, unilateral symptoms, and a negative Phalen sign were predictive of better outcomes.

There are articles about certain exercises for CTS, but in my opinion carpal tunnel syndrome is an overuse problem of the hands and no specific therapeutic exercises are helpful or should be advised.

In 2013 Peters, et al, writing for the *Cochrane Neuromuscular Disease Group* on "Rehabilitation following carpal tunnel release" stated:

...we found limited and low-quality evidence for the benefit of the reviewed treatments including: immobilization with a wrist orthosis (splint), dressings used post surgery, exercise, cold and ice therapy, different types of hand rehabilitation in combination, laser therapy, electrical treatments, scar desensitization...

<u>Medication</u>

Traditionally nonsteroidal anti-inflammatory medications (NSAIDs) have been prescribed for their anti-inflammatory and analgesic activity although articles supportive of NSAID treatment are nonexistent. Also diuretics like Lasix or hydrochlorothiazide have been prescribed on the unsupported theory that median nerve edema may be treated. However, CTS in not an inflammatory or edematous condition.

The *BMJ Clinical Evidence Handbook* stated: We do not know whether NSAIDs...are effective in treating carpal tunnel syndrome. Diuretics seem unlikely to be beneficial in the treatment of carpal tunnel syndrome.

NICE (National Institute for Health and Care Excellence) giving advice in 2012 to primary care physicians regarding treatment of CTS stated: "Do not recommend the use of nonsterioidal anti-inflammatory drugs or diuretic medication."

Short doses of oral cortisone, like Medrol Dosepak or a week of prednisone 20 mg tid for 7 days are reported to provide brief, but not long-lasting therapy. Since CTS causes median nerve damage, a drug that works on neurogenic pain, such as Neurontin (gabapentin) is a more logical drug choice.

Literature Review

Duman, et al, wrote in the *Journal of Clinical Rheumatology* in 2008 on "Assessment of the efficacy of Gabapentin in Carpal Tunnel Syndrome." This was a prospective clinical trial with 3 months follow-up. Twenty-one patients diagnosed with CTS were given an initial gabapentin dosage of 600 mg/day and increased until satisfactory pain control was achieved. This was a clinical assessment study with no EDX testing. A method of statistical study of pain scores was used and the patients were followed for 3 months. The mean gabapentin dose was 648 mg/day. Two patients dropped out of the study. Improvements in pain intensities, numbness severity, and sleep quality were statistically significant. Duman, et al, stated:

> To our knowledge, this is the first prospective clinical trial investigating the efficacy of gabapentin in CTS. Within the limitations of the current study, preliminary results of our clinical experience suggest that gabapentin might have beneficial effects in the management of refractory symptoms of CTS.

Hui, et al, wrote in the *European Journal of Neurology* in 2010 on "Gabapentin for the treatment of carpal tunnel syndrome: a randomized controlled trial." This was a randomized, double-blinded placebo-controlled trial with the diagnosis made clinically and by EDX studies. Patients were randomly assigned to an active group (71 patients) receiving gabapentin (starting dose 300 mg to a target dose of 900 mg) or placebo (69). By 8 weeks the mean reduction in symptom severity of patients on gabapentin was not significant when compared with placebo. Hui, et al, stated "Gabapentin did not produce a significant reduction in symptom severity compared with placebo over an eight-week period."

Erdemoglu writing in *Neurol India* in 2009 on "The efficacy and safety of gabapentin in carpal tunnel syndrome" studied 41 patients with idiopathic CTS. Symptom and functional status were studied before and at 1, 3, and 6 months of treatment. A median dose of 1800 mg was used and results were a 40% reduction in symptom and functional status. Erdemoglu concluded that "Gabapentin was found to be partially effective and safe in symptomatic treatment of CTS patients."

Comment. Hui, et al, found little effect with gabapentin in lower doses, but higher doses gave adequate pain relief.

<u>Splinting</u>

Splinting the hand in a neutral position at night or during daily activities provides some relief for symptoms of CTS. This involves wearing a loose-fitting splint which immobilizes the wrist. Splints may be purchased commonly in drugstores. The purpose of the splint is to hold the wrist in a neutral position, so it need not be tight. Common splints are made of cotton fabric with metal stays and Velcro snaps. They should go on like a glove and immobilize the wrist.

Splinting at night helps when the hand gets bent in flexed positions and when the pressure in the carpal tunnel has been observed to increase. The pressure in the tunnel increases overnight due to mild edema and decreased venous return from muscular inactivity. Splinting may help significantly after just a few days. Many persons with mild CTS wear their splints for a few nights or a few weeks when their symptoms trouble them after some activity such as painting the garage or clipping the weeds in the yard. Many patients, in offices all over America, wear their splints during the day but not at night. Splinting should always be done at night and if it helps, then splinting may be done at work or during daytime activities. The splints should be used for weeks to months depending on the severity of the problem.

Literature Review

Goodman and Gilliatt wrote in the *Annals of Physical Medicine* in 1962 on "The Effect of Treatment On Median Nerve Conduction In Patients With the Carpal Tunnel Syndrome." The authors stated:

Although the results of splinting were variable and often disappointing compared with the uniformly good results of surgery, several points of interest have emerged. In the first place, our results confirm the observations of Heathfield K.W..(Acroparaesthesiae and the carpal-tunnel syndrome. *Lancet.*1957 Oct 5;273(6997):663–666) that some patients with carpal tunnel syndrome do obtain symptomatic relief with this form of treatment. This occurred in a much higher proportion of Heathfield's cases than our own, a difference which is almost certainly explained by the fact that Heathfield's series contained only mildly affected patients, those with thenar wasting or persistent sensory loss being rejected.

Splinting the wrist was tried in 25 cases and motor conduction was examined repeatedly during treatment for periods up to two years. Results were variable, and in some patients abnormalities of conduction were seen to increase during the course of treatment.

Walker, et al, wrote in the *Archives of Physical Medicine and Rehabilitation* in 2000 on "Neutral wrist splinting in carpal tunnel syndrome: A comparison of night-only versus full-time wear." Seventeen outpatients from the authors' EMG lab were instructed to wear thermoplastic, custom-molded neutral wrist splints in two groups: nighttime use only or full time. After 6 weeks all the subjects improved in assessment of distal sensory latency, symptom severity, and functional deficits. The authors concluded:

> This study provides added scientific evidence to support the efficacy of neutral wrist splints in CTS and suggests that physiologic improvement is best with full-time splint wear instructions.

Gerritsen, et al, wrote in the *JAMA* in 2002 on "Splinting vs Surgery in the Treatment of Carpal Tunnel Syndrome A randomized controlled trial." The objective of the study was to compare the short-term and long-term efficacy of splinting and surgery for relieving the symptoms of CTS. A randomized controlled trial at 13 neurological outpatient clinics in the Netherlands studied 176 patients with clinically and electrophysiologically confirmed idiopathic CTS were assigned to wrist splinting during the night for 6 weeks (89 patients) or open carpal tunnel release (87 patients). One hundred forty-seven patients (87%) completed the final follow-up assessment 18 months after randomization. Outcome measures were general improvement, number of nights waking up due to symptoms, and severity of symptoms. Surgery was more effective than splinting on all outcome measures. The success rates after 3 months were 80% for the surgery group (61/68 patients) and 54% for the splinting group (46/86 patients). After 18 months, the success rates increased to 90% for the surgery group vs 75% for the splinting group. However, by that time 41% of patients in the splint group had also received the surgery treatment. Gerritsen, et al, concluded:

> Treatment with open carpal tunnel release surgery resulted in better outcomes than treatment with wrist splinting for patients with CTS.

Werner, et al, wrote "Randomized controlled trial of nocturnal splinting for active workers with symptoms of carpal tunnel syndrome" in 2005 in *Arch Phys Med Rehabil*. The authors studied whether nocturnal splinting of workers at a Midwestern auto assembly plant with symptoms of CTS would improve. The treatment group received customized wrist splints which were worn at night for 6 weeks. The results were that "the splinted group, unlike controls, had a significant reduction in wrist, hand, and/or finger discomfort…which was maintained at 12 months."

De Angelis, et al, writing in *Acta Neurol Scand* in 2009 on "Efficacy of a soft hand brace and a wrist splint for carpal tunnel syndrome: A randomized controlled study" reported on 120 patients for 3 months with EDX confirmed CTS. Some patients continued splinting until the 9-month follow-up evaluation. Both groups found significant relief of symptoms at 3 months, less relief at 9 months, and no change in EDX parameters at any point. At 9 months the rigid brace relieved pain better than the soft brace did.

This article was reviewed in *Journal Watch Neurology* and the editor commented on the interesting aspects of the trial being:

the lack of effect on electrophysiology, the relief of symptoms primarily when the splint was being used (during the first 3 months), and the great diminishment of relief at 9 months (6 months after officially discontinuing splint wear).

These findings add further circumstantial evidence to support the theory that idiopathic median nerve dysfunction at the carpal tunnel is largely an inherent (genetic), eventually bilateral, and inevitably but slowly progressive disease for which splint treatment is only palliative. Despite these findings, we will not change our practice of recommending ongoing night-time wrist splinting for symptom control.

Feng and Gao wrote in *Zhongguo Xiu Fu Chong Jian Wai Ke Za Zhi* in 2011 on "Research progress of treatment of carpal tunnel syndrome." This was a review of recent literature concerning the treatment method of CTS. The authors reported that "Wrist splinting and local steroid injection are effective in patients with mild to moderate CTS in the short-term, however, patients with recurrent CTS have to accept surgical treatment."

Page, et al, writing in the *Cochrane Database Syst Rev* in 2012 on "Splinting for carpal tunnel syndrome" compared the effectiveness of splinting with no treatment, placebo, or another non-surgical intervention. The authors searched the Cochrane Neuromuscular Disease Group Specialized Register, CENTRAL, NHSEED and DARE, MEDLINE, EMBASE, and CINAHL. They excluded studies comparing splinting with surgical treatment. The authors concluded after this literature review that:

Overall, there is limited evidence that a splint worn at night is more effective than no treatment in the short term, but there is insufficient evidence regarding the effectiveness and safety of one splint design or wearing regimen over others, and of splint over other non-surgical interventions for CTS. More research is needed on the long-term effects of this intervention for CTS.

Hall, et al, wrote in 2013 in the *Am J Occup Ther* on "Investigating the effectiveness of full-time wrist splinting and education in the treatment of carpal tunnel syndrome: a randomized controlled trial." This was a study of hospital surgical wait list patients assigned randomly to a control and an intervention group. The intervention consisted of wearing a wrist support splint for 8 weeks and receiving a formal education program on patients with CTS. Significant improvements in measures of symptom severity and functional status occurred in the intervention group only. The authors stated that "This conservative CTS treatment program conducted by occupational therapists can improve symptoms and hand function in CTS patients."

Matzon, et al, wrote in *Orthopedics* in 2013 "Adherence to the American Academy of Orthopedic Surgeons (AAOS) upper extremity clinical practice guidelines." This was an email survey of members of the American Society for Surgery of the Hand (ASSH) to determine adherence to previously published clinical practice guidelines. Overall, 469 responses were obtained for a response rate of 32%. Ninety eight percent of ASSH members advised nighttime splinting in the non-operative treatment of CTS.

Povlsen, et al, wrote in *J Plast Surg Hand Surg* in 2014 on "Long-term result and patient reported outcome of wrist splint treatment for Carpal Tunnel Syndrome." Seventy-five patients referred to a specialist hand clinic with CTS were given night wrist splint treatment for 3 months. Fifty-two patients did not wish to have surgery after wrist splint treatment and were followed a further 33 months. Of the patients who completed the follow-up questionaire 33 months after conservative management, 43% were successfully treated with splinting alone. Patients successfully treated with wrist splinting alone had a higher level of satisfaction compared to patients who failed wrist splint treatment or had surgical decompression. The authors thought the results: "reinforced wrist splinting as a first-line treatment in the Primary Care setting."

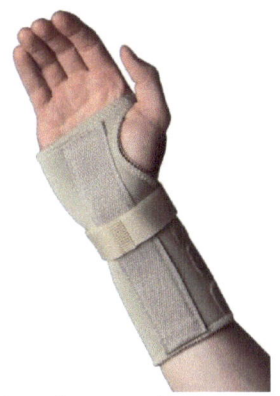

Hand Splint For CTS

Alternative Treatment

In 2003 O'Connor, et al, wrote for the *Cochrane Neuromuscular Disease Group* on "Non-surgical treatment (other than steroid injection) for carpal tunnel syndrome." The authors stated:

> Two trials involving 105 people compared ergonomic keyboards versus control and demonstrated equivocal results for pain and function. Trials of magnet therapy, laser acupuncture, exercise or chiropractic care did not demonstrate symptom benefit when compared to placebo or control.

Chapter 9 Cortisone Injection

This involves injection of cortisone, usually methylprednisolone, by a small (27 gauge) needle through the skin at the first crease of the wrist, through the transverse carpal ligament, and directly into the carpal tunnel. Cortisone injection can shrink the swollen median nerve and relieve pressure. It may give relief in more than 75% of CTS patients but there may be a transient increase in pain for a day or two after the injection. Wrist carpal tunnel injections may cause overlying skin change. Unfortunately, in many cases, the relief is temporary and, in that situation, the injection may be repeated, usually at monthly intervals for up to a total of three injections. The injection is like getting a shot of cortisone for tennis elbow or bursitis and is usually nothing significant. The wrist injection doesn't have generalized or systemic effect. Sometimes during the injection if the needle lies too near the nerve, the patient may experience transient symptoms of numbness but repositioning the needle during the injection will avoid this. Also, multiple injections may be associated with tendon rupture.

Literature Review

Goodman and Foster writing in the *British Association of Physical Medicine* in 1962 on "Effect of local corticosteroid injection on median nerve conduction in carpal tunnel syndrome." The authors reported the effects of local corticosteroid injection on median nerve conduction in 23 patients with CTS. The injections gave relief of symptoms and improved distal motor median latencies with relapses occurring between 9 and 15 months after injection. Goodman and Foster suggested "corticosteroid injection for CTS in pregnancy in whom spontaneous improvement may be expected after parturition." They also suggested similar treatment for patients with myxedema (British term for hypothyroidism), giving relief with injection until myxedema itself was controlled by medical treatment and in patients with advanced age, cardiac, or pulmonary conditions which would preclude surgery.

Paddu, et al, presented a poster for the 1996 annual AAEM meeting entitled: "A Pilot Investigation to Develop Instrumentation for The Efficacy of Corticosteroid Injection For Carpal Tunnel Syndrome: A Single-Blinded Study." The authors developed a questionaire to evaluate subjective symptoms and standardized isometric testing with hand grasp and pinch gauge. Eight female patients with EDX confirmed CTS were given 1cc (4mg) dexamethasone and ¼ cc of lidocaine at the first volar wrist crease into the carpal tunnel. The patients were evaluated at entrance and at 3 months. The result was that grip strength improved in 6/8 patients and subjective improvement was noted in seven; one patient was unchanged. Paddu stated:

> We conclude that steroid injection has a role in alleviating symptoms of CTS with significant subjective and objective improvement

noted at 3 months with objective instrumentation.

Amirjani et al, writing in *Muscle & Nerve* in 2009 on "Corticosteroid Iontophoresis to Treat Carpal Tunnel Syndrome: Double-Blind Randomized Controlled Trial" stated that:

> Local injection of 40 mg of methylprednisolone into the carpal tunnel in mild CTS significantly reduces the symptoms in 80% of patients for at least 16 months and normalizes EDX parameters in 50 % of the subjects for 12 months after treatment. Corticosteroid Iontophoresis with 0.4% dexamethasone is not effective in the treatment of mild to moderate CTS.

Marshall, et al, writing for the *Cochrane Neuromuscular Disease Group* in 2007 on "Local corticosteroid injection for carpal tunnel syndrome" evaluated the effectiveness of local corticosteroid injection for carpal tunnel syndrome versus placebo injection or other non-surgical interventions. They performed a literature search of MEDLINE, EMBASE, CINAHL, and the Cochrane Neuromuscular Disease Group Trials register and found 12 studies with 671 participants. The authors concluded:

> Local corticosteroid injection is a common non-surgical treatment for carpal tunnel syndrome. Other non-surgical treatments include the use of wrist splint splints, ultrasound, and

oral anti-inflammatory agents. Surgical intervention is also known to be effective. This systematic review confirmed the effectiveness of local corticosteroid injection for relief of symptoms for severe carpal tunnel syndrome up to one month after injection. Local corticosteroid injection provides significantly greater clinical improvement compared to oral corticosteroid up to three months after treatment. Two injections of local corticosteroid do not provide significant further clinical improvement of symptoms. Further research is required to determine length of benefit of local corticosteroid injection and benefit for mild and moderate carpal tunnel syndrome.

The editors of the *BMJ Clinical Evidence Handbook* in 2008 writing on CTS stated:

Corticosteroid treatment (either local injection or systemic) appears to be beneficial in treating carpal tunnel syndrome, although the evidence suggests that there is greater improvement in long-term outcomes with local injections compared with systemic administration.

Cartwright, et al, writing in *Muscle & Nerve* in 2009 on "Median nerve changes following steroid injection for carpal tunnel syndrome" reported a decrease in the median nerve cross-sectional area on ultrasound along with changes in nerve mobility, echogenicity, and vascularity which occurred within 1 week of steroid injection. These changes were of greater statistical significance than changes in NCSs.

Meys, et al, wrote in *Muscle & Nerve* in 2011 on "Prognostic factors in carpal tunnel syndrome treated with a corticosteroid injection." They studied 113 patients who received injection for CTS who were followed with clinical, electrophysiological, and ultrasonographic tests at baseline, 1, 3, 6, and 12 months. The primary outcome measure for success was no need for further treatment, e.g. surgery. After 1 month most patients improved, but after 12 months 67.4% had surgery. Patients with a successful outcome had a lower median nerve ultrasonographic cross-sectional area at the pisiform bone, a lower swelling ratio, and a lower symptom severity score. They concluded that:

> less pronounced median nerve swelling measured by ultrasonography may indicate a less severe stage of CTS, which is more likely to respond to treatment with a corticosteroid injection.

Atroshi, et al, wrote in the *Annals of Internal Medicine* in 2013 on "Methylprednisolone Injections for the Carpal Tunnel Syndrome: A Randomized, Placebo-Controlled Trial." This was a study of the efficacy of local methylprednisolone injections in CTS conducted at an orthopedic regional referral department in Sweden. Three groups of 37 patients received 80 mg methylprednisolone, 40 mg methylprednisolone, or placebo. The primary end points were the change in CTS symptoms severity scores at 10 weeks (range, 1 to 5) and rate of surgery at 1 year. The results were:

improvement in CTS symptom severity scores at 10 weeks was greater in patients who received 80 mg of methylprednisolone than those who received placebo.

Patients who received 80 mg of methylprednisolone were less likely to have surgery. This was a one center study and all patients had previously failed wrist splinting. The conclusion was:

Methylprednisolone injections for CTS have significant benefits in relieving symptoms at 10 weeks and reducing the rate of surgery 1 year after treatment, but ¾ patients had surgery within 1 year.

Verdugo, et al, writing in 2008 in the *Cochrane Neuromuscular Disease Group* on "Surgical versus non-surgical treatment for carpal tunnel syndrome" compared the efficacy of surgical treatment of carpal tunnel syndrome with non-surgical treatment. Verdugo, et al, concluded:

Surgical treatment of carpal tunnel syndrome relieves symptoms significantly better than splinting. Further research is needed to discover whether this conclusion applies to people with mild symptoms and whether surgical treatment is better than steroid injection.

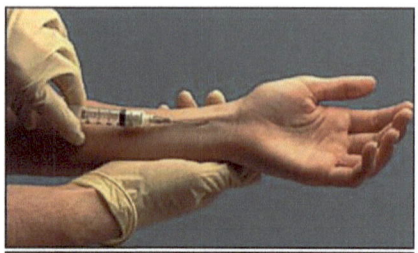

Cortisone Injection

Chapter 10 Surgery

If conservative management fails, or if clinical and electrophysiological assessment indicates, then surgery should be considered. Carpal tunnel surgery is one of the most common and successful of all surgeries.

Success rate

Surgery for CTS may provide good results for about 81% of patients although about 9% of patients report that they are unchanged or worse after surgery. There is a wide variation in reported success rates, ranging from 27% to 100%. The literature suggests that some surgeons through good case selection and technical excellence achieve much better than average results. Misdiagnosis and surgical errors are the principal causes of surgical failure. The success rate of surgery performed on purely clinical grounds in the presence of normal nerve conduction studies (NCS) is noticeably lower than that of similar operations performed when NCS are abnormal. Many patients require surgery on both hands. Older age patients in general and patients with worse preoperative neurologic dysfunction (thenar atrophy, median digit sensory loss for pin) are not as likely as younger patients to have a good surgical outcome.

Types of surgery

Open release surgery, the traditional procedure used to correct carpal tunnel syndrome, consists of making an incision up to 3 cm in the wrist and then cutting the carpal ligament to enlarge the carpal tunnel. The procedure is generally done under local anesthesia on an outpatient basis, unless there are unusual medical considerations.

Endoscopic surgery may allow faster functional recovery and less postoperative discomfort than traditional open release surgery. The surgeon makes two incisions (about 1-1/2 cm each) in the wrist and palm, inserts a camera attached to a tube, observes the tissue on a screen, and cuts the carpal ligament. This two-portal endoscopic surgery, generally performed under local anesthesia, is effective and minimizes scarring and scar tenderness, if any. Single portal endoscopic surgery for carpal tunnel syndrome is also available and can result in less postoperative pain and a minimal scar. It generally allows individuals to resume some normal activities in a short period of time. A smaller scar in the palm area may allow less pain in the postoperative period. However, endoscopic surgery is generally more expensive than open release surgery. Some surgeons feel that damage to the median nerve is less likely with an open release approach because of direct visualization of the transverse carpal ligament.

Literature Review

Astroski, et al, wrote in the *BMJ* in 2006 on "Outcomes of endoscopic surgery compared with open surgery for carpal tunnel syndrome among employed patients: randomized controlled trial." The authors compared result of surgery for CTS in 128 patients with clinically diagnosed and electrophysiologically confirmed idiopathic carpal tunnel syndrome. Sixty-three patients had endoscopic surgery and 65 had open surgery. The primary outcome was severity of postoperative pain in the scar and proximal palm and the degree to which pain or tenderness limits activities. This was rated on a numerical scale. Astroski, et al, reported:

> Pain in the scar or proximal palm was less prevalent or severe after endoscopic surgery than after open surgery, but the differences were generally small.
>
> The median length of work absence after surgery was 28 days in both groups.
>
> In carpal tunnel syndrome, endoscopic surgery was associated with less postoperative pain than open surgery, but the small size of the benefit and similarity in other outcomes make its cost effectiveness uncertain.

Scholten, et al, wrote for the *Cochrane Neuromuscular Disease Group* in 2007 "Surgical treatment options for carpal tunnel syndrome." The objectives were to "compare the efficacy of the various surgical techniques in relieving symptoms and promoting return to work or activities of daily living and to compare the occurrence of side-effects and complications in patients suffering from carpal tunnel syndrome." The authors purused computer-aided searches of MEDLINE, EMBASE, the Cochrane Neuromuscular Disease Group Trials Register, and the Cochrane library. Thirty-three studies were included in the review and the authors stated:

Severe cases are generally treated surgically. Current evidence from randomized controlled trials showed that none of the alternatives to standard open carpal tunnel release seem to offer better relief from symptoms in the short- or long-term, although a special type of operation (endoscopic carpal tunnel release) seems to enable people to return to their work or daily activities sooner (on average approximately a week).

Kohanzadeh, et al, wrote in *Hand* (N Y) in 2012 on "Outcomes of open and endoscopic carpal tunnel release: a meta-analysis." This was a meta-analysis of retrospective series of carpal tunnel release including over 20 patients and measuring 6 of 9 outcome measures such as paresthesia relief, scar tenderness, two-point discrimination, thenar muscle weakness, monofilament testing, return to work time, grip and pinch strength, and complications. Kohanzadeh reported:

Endoscopic carpal tunnel approach showed statistically superior outcomes in 8 of the 9 categories investigated. Only in the category of complications (mean occurrence of 1.2% in the open release versus 2.2% in the endoscopic release group) was the endoscopic group inferior.

This suggests that the endoscopic release is superior to the open release, particularly in experienced hands.

Who should be operated?

Surgery is more effective for patients with moderate to severe carpal tunnel syndrome, those over age 50, those with symptoms of 10 months or longer, those with continual numbness, and those with thumb base atrophy. It is the treatment of choice for patients with post-fracture, polyneuropathy, or arthritic induced nerve damage. It is also the only treatment that will allow some patients to return to work at a job that requires continual stress of the median nerve in the carpal tunnel. One lay misperception regarding carpal tunnel syndrome is that if you have it, then you automatically need surgical treatment; some may need surgery, others do well with conservative treatment.

Literature review

Goodman and Gilliat writing in the *Annals of Physical Medicine* in 1962 in their landmark article on "The Effect of Treatment On Median Nerve Conduction In Patients With The Carpal Tunnel Syndrome" stated:

However, these points do not detract from the general conclusion that an adequate operation is such a highly satisfactory procedure in the carpal tunnel syndrome that for all practical purposes it constitutes a curative treatment for this condition.

The clinical results of surgery were satisfactory in all cases, relief of pain being rapid and complete.

In our surgical series it is extremely gratifying that operation had such a satisfactory result in relieving symptoms and reversing disordered nerve function. So far as motor conduction is concerned, every patient came back into the normal range, although after two years most of the cases in the severe group still showed latencies slightly above the normal mean.

Surgical division of the anterior carpal ligament was carried out in 23 cases. Serial examinations of motor conduction for up to two years after operation showed satisfactory recovery of conduction in all cases, the recovery time depending on the severity of the initial lesion.

Cseuz, et al, writing in *Mayo Clin Proc* in 1966 on "Long-Term Results Of Operation For Carpal Tunnel Syndrome" studied 313 patients (75 men and 238 women) seen at the Mayo Clinic who had a final diagnosis of CTS, an EMG examination, and surgical decompression of the median nerve. The authors stated:

In many cases the operative scar was sensitive for years after operation.

The present study indicates that the long-term postoperative results are very gratifying. After an average follow-up of 3 years and a maximal follow-up of 8 years, 81% of the 313 patients reported complete or near complete recovery, and an additional 10% claimed improvement.

Patients who did not benefit from the operation made up 9% of our series.

It was found that advanced aged did not preclude good post-operative results. However, good results were not obtained as frequently in older patients as they were in younger patients.

No evidence was found that duration of symptoms affected surgical success.

The electromyogram proved to be highly valuable in the diagnostic evaluation of CTS, but if failed to provide information useful in predicting surgical success.

The presence of advanced diabetes and rheumatoid arthritis in patients with CTS has previously made us hesitant to predict lasting relief of symptoms postoperatively. The current results, however, suggest that excessive concern in this regard is not warranted.

The information gathered in this investigation suggests that a patient with carpal tunnel syndrome can be of advanced age, can have had his symptoms for many years, can reveal impairment of neurologic function, can show marked electromyographic abnormalities, and can be afflicted with such conditions as diabetes and rheumatoid arthritis and still have a good chance to be completely relieved of his symptoms by surgical decompression of the median nerve.

Failure of the patient to benefit from operation occurred in 1 of every 10 cases, but a consistent cause for this was not found.

Harris, et al, wrote in *The Journal of Bone and Joint Surgery* in 1979 on "The Surgical Treatment of the Carpal Tunnel Syndrome Correlated with Preoperative Nerve Conduction Studies." This was a study of 124 cases (101 patients) with CTS diagnosed clinically and by nerve conduction studies. The authors found that:

Retrospective analysis of the series suggests that nerve conduction studies can be used as a prognostic factor. Those patients with motor abnormalities appeared to have a more favorable result than those with only sensory abnormalities.

Clayburgh, et al, wrote in *The Journal of Hand Surgery* in 1987 on "Carpal tunnel release in patients with diffuse peripheral neuropathy." The authors stated:

Sixty carpal tunnel decompressions were performed in 44 patients with combined carpal tunnel syndrome and peripheral neuropathy. Symptomatic improvement was obtained in 92% of the patients and complete relief of symptoms in 72%. We conclude that peripheral neuropathy is not a contraindication to carpal tunnel decompression.

The American Academy of Orthopedic Surgeons published "AAOS Clinical guidelines on the Treatment of Carpal tunnel syndrome" in *AAOS Now* in 2008. The editors stated:

A course of nonoperative treatment is an option in patients diagnosed with carpal tunnel syndrome. Early surgery is an option when there is clinical evidence of median nerve denervation or the patient elects to proceed directly to surgical treatment.

We do not have sufficient evidence to provide specific treatment recommendations for carpal tunnel syndrome when found in association with the following conditions: diabetes mellitus, coexistent cervical radiculopathy, hypothyroidism, polyneuropathy, pregnancy, rheumatoid arthritis, and carpal tunnel syndrome in the workplace.

Local steroid injection or splinting is suggested when treating patients with carpal tunnel syndrome, before considering surgery.

Oral steroids or ultrasound are options when treating patients with carpal tunnel syndrome.

We recommend carpal tunnel release as treatment for carpal tunnel syndrome.

The following treatments carry no recommendation for or against their use: activity modifications, acupuncture, cognitive behavioral therapy, cold laser, diuretics, exercise, electric stimulation, fitness, Graston instrument, Iontophoresis, laser, stretching, massage therapy, magnet therapy, manipulation, medications (including anticonvulsants, antidepressants, and Nonsteroidal anti-inflammatory drugs [NSAIDS]), nutritional supplements, phonophoresis, smoking cessation, systemic steroid injection, therapeutic touch, vitamin V6 (pyridoxine), weight reduction, yoga.

We recommend surgical treatment of carpal tunnel syndrome by complete division of the flexor retinaculum regardless of the specific surgical technique.

We suggest that the wrist not
be immobilized postoperatively after
routine carpal tunnel surgery.
We make no recommendations
for or against the use of postoperative
rehabilitation.

In 2008 the editors of *BMJ* writing on
treatment of Carpal Tunnel Syndrome stated:
Surgery seems to improve
clinical outcomes compared with wrist
splints, but is not as effective as local
corticosteroid injections.

Both endoscopic and open
carpal tunnel release seem to improve
symptoms, although the data are
unclear as to which is more beneficial.
Both are associated with several
adverse effects.

Thomsen, et al, wrote in the *J Hand Surg Am*
in 2014 on "Carpal tunnel release in patients with
diabetes: a 5-year follow-up with matched controls."
The purpose of this study was to compare clinical
outcomes 5 years after carpal tunnel release among
patients with and without diabetes. In a prospective
series 35 patients with diabetes were age and sex-
matched with 31 control patients without diabetes.
Thomsen, et al, reported:
Long-term improvement in
patients with diabetes remained after
carpal tunnel release to the same extent
as for patients without diabetes.
Furthermore, improvement in cold
intolerance in patients with diabetes

suggests the potential for the long-term regeneration of small nerve fibers.

Post-operative recovery

Although symptoms may be relieved immediately after surgery, full recovery from carpal tunnel surgery can take months. Some patients may have infection, nerve damage, stiffness, and pain at the site of the scar. Anti-inflammatory medications like Advil (ibuprofen) should be stopped before surgery but aspirin may be used safely through surgery. Occasionally the wrist loses strength because the carpal ligament is cut. Some patients may need to adjust job duties or even change jobs after recovery from surgery.

Recurrence of CTS

Recurrence of carpal tunnel syndrome following treatment is rare. The majority of patients recover completely. Cause of recurrence is poorly understood, and likely multifactorial but incomplete severance of the transverse carpal ligament is the most common cause.

Causes of surgical error

The most common surgical error is failure to completely divide the transverse carpal ligament. This issue sparks the differences between proponents of open release CTS surgery as opposed to endoscopic surgery. The incidence of failure to divide the transverse carpal ligament is higher with endoscopic surgery because the ligament is not as well visualized with the endoscopic technique. Injuries to the recurrent motor and palmar cutaneous branches of the median nerve are well recognized and both median and ulnar nerve trunk lacerations have been reported.

Post-surgery complications

Possible post-surgery problems include: wound infections, vascular injuries to the superficial palmar arch, painful scar formation, and complex regional pain syndrome. The combined incidence of these problems should result in no more than 1-2% long-term disability after carpal tunnel surgery. After successful decompression that relieved symptoms for some time, true recurrence of CTS is a rare event.

Causes of failed carpal tunnel release

Numbness, pain, and weakness in the hand can be caused by other syndromes. Witt and Stevens wrote in the *Mayo Clinic Proceedings* in 2000 on "Neurologic Disorders masquerading as Carpal Tunnel Syndrome: 12 Cases of Failed Carpal Tunnel Release." After further assessment of these 12 cases Witt and Stevens stated:

Final diagnoses included polyneuropathy, radiculopathy, motor neuron disease, spondylotic myelopathy, syringomyelia, and multiple sclerosis.

Witt and Stevens found that one of their 12 cases with no improvement after surgical release had no confirmatory preoperative EMG.

Among the EMGs, errors were as follows: inadequate NCS to identify polyneuropathy (such as no radial or ulnar studies), inadequate needle EMG to exclude radiculopathy, no temperature control, failure to report amplitude data, failure to report normal reference values, diagnosis of CTS based solely on motor delay with normal results of sensory studies, failure to explain denervation in nonmedian innervated muscles, diagnosis of multiple mononeuropathies (such as median and ulnar) in cases of polyneuropathy. Clinical pitfalls included failure to observe nonmedian neurologic deficits, failure to elicit signs of a central disorder, diagnosing "pure motor CTS" in the absence of sensory symptoms, and diagnosing CTS when the examination or EMG findings suggested a different disorder.

Extreme Carpal Tunnel Syndrome

Capasso, et al, wrote in 2009 in *Muscle & Nerve* on "Management of Extreme Carpal Tunnel Syndrome: Evidence From a Long-Term Follow-up Study." The authors defined "extreme carpal tunnel syndrome" as: severe thenar atrophy, plegia of the abductor pollicis brevis, fixed sensory deficit in the median nerve distribution, and absence of median motor and sensory responses on electrophysiological examination. Capasso, et al, studied 24 patients with idiopathic extreme CTS, 9 untreated, 3 with conservative management. At follow-up of these patients none showed objective or electrophysiological improvement, and all but 1 still reported positive symptoms. However, 12 patients

(14 hands) who had surgery showed resolution of positive symptoms in all but 1 hand, reappearance of motor compound muscle action potentials, reappearance of sensory nerve action potentials in all but 1, improvement of APB strength to grade 4 or 5 on the Medical Research Council scale in 11 hands; and resolution of hypesthesia in 1 hand. Six of 13 patients with non-idiopathic extreme CTS were operated. Of the 6, no or poor reinnervation was found in 3 patients, restoration of nerve responses and normal APB strength but no relief from pain and/or paresthesia in 2, and full recovery in 1. The authors stressed that:

> If untreated, extreme CTS is an irreversible condition. Although the outcome is considered to be disappointing in such cases, carpal tunnel release provides long-term relief, significant sensorimotor reinnervation, and improvement of motor deficit in most patients.

> It should be considered to be the first-choice treatment for idiopathic extreme CTS. Associated diseases do not necessarily imply a poor surgical outcome.

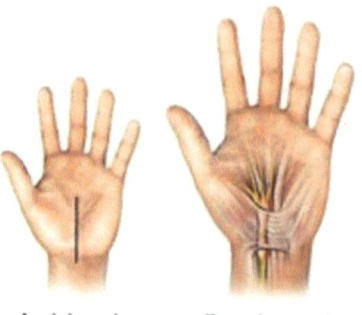
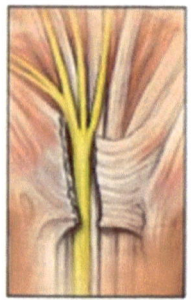

Incision site   Carpal tunnel   Median nerve
released

Open Surgery For CTS

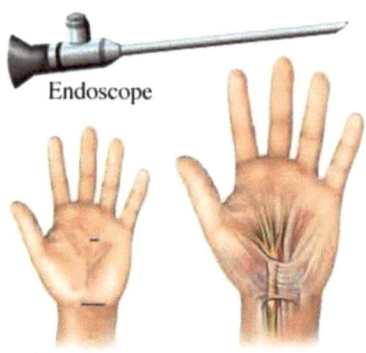
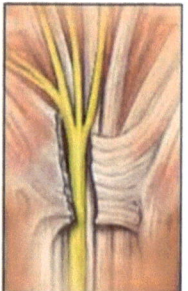

Endoscope

Portal sites   Carpal tunnel   Median nerve
for endoscope   released

Endoscopic Surgery For CTS

Natural history of CTS

To compare various treatments of CTS such as splinting, cortisone injection, or surgery, it is important to consider the natural history of untreated idiopathic CTS. The available studies here are limited.

Tachibana, et al, wrote in 1979 in *Acta Neurologica Scand* on "Prognosis in Carpal Tunnel

Syndrome: A Comparison Between The Natural History and Operative Treatment." The authors studied 172 (15 male and 157 female cases) of CTS to follow the natural course of this disorder. The group that was treated conservatively or given no treatment at all consisted of 161 patients whom the authors contacted for follow-up information. Of this group 119 (74%) responded the final report consisted of the 119 untreated and 15 operated cases comparing the difference in sensory conduction velocities of the median nerve studied antidromically from wrist to finger and distal motor latencies at the wrist to APB. There was no significant NCS difference between those patients whose symptoms cured spontaneously (56) and those patients whose symptoms still remained (112). Also there was no significant difference in the sensory and motor conduction velocities between the first and last examination (50). In contrast, in the group of operative treatment (15), there was statistically significant improvement between pre-and post-operative sensory and motor velocities.

Padua, et al, wrote in *Neurology* in 2001 on "Multiperspective follow-up of untreated carpal tunnel syndrome: a multicenter study." The objective of this study was to assess the course of untreated carpal tunnel syndrome. The Italian CTS Study Group prospectively followed up 441 affected hands with idiopathic CTS, 21% improved over 10-15 months of follow-up without active intervention, although 68% of the patients made efforts to reduce occupational and recreational hand stress and 32% changed either hobby or work. CTS measurements

improved in patients with more severe initial
impairment whereas they worsened in patients with
milder initial impairment. Positive prognostic factors
were short duration of symptoms, younger age,
unilateral CTS involvement, and a negative Phalen
sign. The authors' conclusion was that "Some
patients with CTS improve spontaneously without
surgical treatment."

      Comment. To be fair, Padua's patients did
have some sort of "treatment" which was rest and
change of use of a limb, allowing some recovery. To
state that Padua's patients improved spontaneously is
deceptive because rest and change of use are
conservative treatments.

      Bland wrote in Muscle & Nerve in 2007 on
"Treatment of Carpal Tunnel Syndrome" Bland cited
the Cochrane systemic reviews:

> Although these give a good
> summary of the currently available
> evidence, their predominant
> conclusion is that the evidence for
> most interventions is of very poor
> quality and the way in which they are
> presented does not make it easy to
> advise the individual patient of the
> likely outcomes of the various
> treatment options available.

      He suggested that the treatment options should
be compared with doing nothing and quoted Padua, et
al, (above article) as the best sole source of data on
the natural history of carpal tunnel syndrome and that
"any therapeutic intervention should hope to achieve
a better than 21% improvement rate." Bland stated:

Fifty years after its widespread recognition, a significant minority of patients with carpal tunnel syndrome continue to experience poor outcomes from treatment. Much current treatment is supported by an inadequate or nonexistent evidence base. Surgical decompression, often considered the definitive solution, gives excellent results in only 75% of cases in ordinary practice and leaves 8% of patients worse than previously. The only other interventions that are clearly of benefit are neutral-angle wrist splinting with a success rate of 37% and steroids, which are better given by local injection than as oral treatment. The initial response rate to injection is 70% but there are frequent relapses. Nevertheless, these conservative treatments have a negligible incidence of serious complications and should be used more widely until surgical failures can be reduced to similar levels.

Comment. Bland's statement could be compared with the results of Cseuz, et al, in 1966 who found that "long-term postoperative results were very gratifying," with 81% of patients reporting complete or near complete recovery, an additional 10 % claimed improvement, and 9% who did not benefit. His statement that 8% are worse is not supported by the study by Cseuz, et al. What is stated is that 9%

did not benefit from surgery and in this group, some were patients with unchanged symptoms and others who were worse. Bland's comments are also out of line with Clayburg, et al, in 1987 who operated conceptually a worse group of CTS patients with peripheral neuropathy who had "symptomatic improvement in 92% of patients and complete relief of symptoms in 72%.

Splinting for years and getting repeat injections of cortisone in the wrist, at best temporizes the problem, while the overwhelming majority of patients who have carpal tunnel syndrome and want to finally get it over with, will have carpal tunnel release and enjoy a permanent cure of the condition.

***

About the Author

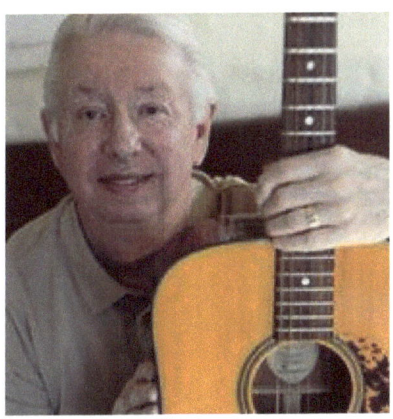

Britt Talley Daniel MD is a retired neurologist from Dallas, Texas. Trained in medicine at the University of Texas Medical Branch in Galveston and in neurology at the Mayo Clinic in Rochester, Minnesota. Dr. Daniel served his country as a staff neurologist LCDR, USNR at Balboa Hospital in San Diego, California during the Vietnam War.

After this he was on the senior staff as a neurologist at Scott and White Clinic in Temple, Texas, and an Associate Professor of Neurology at Texas A&M University Medical School. Moving to Dallas to start a private practice, Dr. Daniel taught at the University of Texas Southwestern Medical School as a Clinical Associate Professor of Neurology.

Currently he is a retired member of the American Academy of Neurology, the American Headache Society, and the American Association of Neuromuscular and Electrodiagnostic Medicine.

Married and with 5 grown children, Dr. Daniel is a lifelong singer and guitarist. He is also the author of 5 medical textbooks:
Migraine
Transient Global Amnesia
The Mini Neurology Series: Volume 1 Migraine,
Volume 2 Carpal Tunnel Syndrome
Volume 3 Panic Disorder
and Volume 4 Essential Tremor.
He has written a transgenerational novel about a medical family from England who relocates to America aboard the haunted Titanic, entitled:
Titanic Answer from the Deep.
He has also written three books from the Mysteries of MacArthur Donne series entitled:
And If Thine Eye Offend Thee
The Case of the Organic Chemist
and The Spanish Flu 1918.
If you read any of my books, please review them on Amazon. I would really appreciate it.
All eBooks and print books are on Amazon.
All books may be found at my author website:
https://www.britttalleydanielmdaauthor.com
Twitter: http://twitter.com/btdaniel
Facebook: http://www.facebook.com/doctormigraine